THE FIFTH TIME IS A
CHARM!!!
WHY I DIDN'T GIVE UP ON
MYSELF!

Before going any further, I have to give a
special thanks to my Rock, my best friend,
my husband, DeWayne. Without him
holding me up, encouraging, believing me,
and having my back each step of the way,
I'm not sure I could have made it this far.
Thank you for loving me and allowing me to
walk through this life by your side.
Thank you for loving me

Mom,

Thank you for loving me before I knew how to love myself. And thank you for being there every day while I've taken on this lifelong fight against heart disease.

To my mother-in-law, Bobbie, thank you for your constant inspiration. You saw that I could help someone else by sharing my story even when I didn't. You encouraged me to continue writing until I perfected my craft and never gave up on my dream.

Before I start, I want to make sure everyone knows that you have to do your part to get stronger and beat heart disease. Yeah, it's always best for you to follow your doctor's orders, but you will still have to do your part. First, you'll need to do your research on diagnosis and the medications they prescribe. After working in pharmacy for 23 years and a non-profit clinic, I see it every day. Day in and day out, I watched most of our doctors get their information by putting your ethnicity, age, and gender into a database with a cited problem to find a result. But what they forget is that patients are human beings, so what worked for their last patient may or may not work for you. Most doctors feel that women complain or exaggerate about our health which I had to go through for years before someone took the time to listen to me. If it were not for me being adamant, I'd be dead.

When I first started my journey with heart disease, I didn't know what to expect. The only experts I knew were doctors. I didn't have anyone to ask what to expect, what can I or do. My mind raced with a million questions running through my mind at one time. I didn't know what to do other than reach to my husband and my Mom.
I'll get more in detail with that as I go on. Just imagine going from thinking you had indigestion, a cold, pleurisy, or a respiratory infection to hearing you need to see a cardiologist and surgery as soon as possible. That's was me 15 years ago.
There's a lot about me that most people don't know or haven't taken the opportunity to get to know. Being a severe patient is one of the most challenging and best things that could have ever happened.

PRESENT-DAY

This surgery was my 5th heart surgery, yes, fifth, and I must say it wasn't anything like the first four. I had to learn to do simple things.
To be precise, let me explain it correctly. My first and second heart surgeries open using the method of sternotomy, which most people are familiar with ere they crack open your sternal cavity or breast bone. My third

heart surgery was a thoracotomy where I was laid on my left side and cracked my side open. The fourth heart surgery Dr. Petracek tried was a new experimental procedure called TVAR when Transcatheter Valve Aortic Replacement. Instead of having the aortic valve replaced, my Tricuspid Valve was replaced. Last but not least, my fifth was another sternotomy. Ughh, it was painful.

Let's start at the beginning. My name is Charnique Rucker. My family and friends call me Niki or Niq. I'm a 40-year-old African American woman, and I was diagnosed with congenital heart disease when I was 25. I never showed any signs until I turned 24. I've endured a lot in a short period, starting with my first surgery until now while I'm recovering from my last heart surgery. I've been struggling, which is probably a strong word, but I've been going back and forth about really writing about my struggles with heart disease. But you know me if I think it will help someone's journey become a little easier.

My struggle

My struggle began when I was 24, almost 25 years old. I kept catching every cold known to humanity. I kept the worst case of chest pain that my doctors kept writing off as acid reflux. I was straight-up miserable. Nobody thought I knew what I was talking about my husband, doctors, friends, or family. They thought I was just a drama queen looking for attention.

At my first appointment with Dr. Ferguson, he placed his stethoscope against my chest and listened to my heart, and within seconds, he asked, "Has anyone ever told me that you have a heart murmur or any heart problem?

Neither c

I was afraid and happy because he took the time to listen to me first, and just like he just about solved my problems.

Over the past 23 years, I worked as a Certified Pharmacy Technician just about everywhere in Memphis. I've been with Christ Community Health Services for the past ten, almost 11 years. I'm mentioning this only to speak of the cardiac patients that I've come across. So many people live with heart disease with absolutely no idea of what's going with them. I think my love for the patients is what I love most. Those who truly live in poverty are most of our patients. They don't have the resources to help themselves or access the information. It's the same cycle they come in to leave out with 12 medications that have nothing to do with the primary reason the patient went into the clinic. I see over and over. It's the way of the medical field. The doctors only give you enough to have you coming back in with the same complaint and another issue. I tell everyone you have to be adamant about your health. There's a quota they must meet monthly by them. Even though they were only dealing with a fraction of what I was going through, they'd give advice. I passed and shared a lot of struggles with them. One question that never gets old.

"Why are you still working and not at home collecting social security and disability"? My response has always been the same. With a smile, I'd say it's because I can't and won't give up on Charnique. Plain and simple right, I'm just not like most people, giving up. It's not in me, so I keep trying, and I keep pushing.

SURGERY # 1

Let's take a step back to 2004, when I first started having chest pain, numbness, and tingling on my left side. I was in school for nursing around this time, and I'd just begun taking Anatomy and Physiology. Before class let out, I stood in front of a diagram, asking my professor some questions about the muscular system. As I tried to rise from my seat, the sharpest pain I'd ever felt sat my butt back down in that chair. The only thing I could do was hold the center of my chest. There was only one person that noticed was my mother-in-law sitting right across from me. She whispered, "are you okay?

Some kind of a way, I managed to shake my head. As soon as class let out, I headed to the nearest ER at Methodist North Hospital. As usual, they did an EKG and an X-Ray and told me they couldn't find anything. They recommended resting for two to three days and for me to return if my symptoms got worse.

For a little over a year, I went through listening to my doctors insist on my symptoms related to Bronchitis and Upper respiratory infections. I shouldn't have listened to my mother-in-law when she insisted on going to Dr. Thomas Motley and Associates over downtown Methodist Central Hospital. I guess Dr. Motley's office was significant for diabetes, gout, and high blood pressure issues. But not with young patients that have severe heart problems, not so much. They'd prescribed everything from Lortab, Robitussin a/c, Tussionex, omeprazole, Proventil inhalers, Azithromycin, Ceftin, Augmentin, and so much more than that more times than I can count over 12 months.

I should've listened to my Mom when she told me to do my research instead of using somebody else. I battled back and forth with their office for more than a year before giving up and trying someone. At each of my visits, my complaints were different, but the result was always the same. I'd sit in the waiting area for almost two hours, waiting to hear my name. Once in the back, I'd go through standard triage with weight, height, urine sample, medication list, and reason for my visit. After being placed into a room, it's another one to two-hour wait. Either Dr. Motley or his nurse would knock on the door before entering. They'd pretend to listen for about five minutes to tell me I had yet another cold wish that was causing the rattling in my chest.

After working at Walgreens for almost ten years, I cut my hours dropped their

insurance and got new insurance with St. Jude Hospital, where I was full-time.
It wasn't until I passed out outside the IV room one night mid-shift, to be completely honest. I'd just had an appointment with Dr. Thomas Motley's office a few days before to tell me this particular time that I had pleurisy and an upper respiratory infection. Pleurisy causes the inflammation of the tissues that line the lungs and chest cavity.
What the hell?
I'd never heard of it. Again my symptoms were the same. But this time, they said the main complaint was severe chest pain that worsens when breathing.
Nope, it wasn't that either. I was back at square one. It took years for someone to listen to me, even though I was constantly at my doctor's office with one complaint or another.

At my initial visit with Dr. Thomas Ferguson's office with Raleigh-Bartlett Medical Group, he found my problem.

Dr. Ferguson said, has anyone ever told you to have a heart murmur.

Nope, never, am I going to be okay.

He was shocked. You've had it since birth which would make your heart problem is congenital.

Although I'd spoken to the Nurse and explained my chief complaint, he had me give him more detail. I was pissed off. I'd taken so many antibiotics and crap that I didn't need. I could've done more harm than good. The Medical Assistant Jurney set my appointment for Monday, March 15th, 2006, at 9:00 am two weeks away.

At the end of my appointment, he was adamant about keeping the appointment with Sutherland Clinic once his front desk staff schedules it. I did just that. I was scared out of my mind, but I knew I had to do it. I'd taken off a full day because I didn't know what to expect at this visit.

While waiting in the waiting area, I started having chest pain. When I made it to the back to triage, it had intensified. On a scale from one to ten, it was at 9.5. My Nurse, Tiana, stepped out to speak with Dr. Basco as quickly as she could. He came into the room shortly after and asked what exactly that I was feeling. After explaining to him that it was a sharp pain with pressure like somebody was sitting on my chest. He had the Nurse give me Nitro-stat twice. It didn't help at all. I was light-headed like I felt I was about to fall out, but my heart was racing. They checked my vitals, and I heard Dr. Basco yelling out the room for someone to call an ambulance for me. I was surprised to wake up and see his face. He was a resident at the hospital as well, so it wasn't a problem. After he made sure I was stable, he ordered some tests and told me he'd be back before the night's end to check on me. They admitted me for one night, an EKG, x-rays, blood work, and a possible stress test. The hospital didn't get a chance to perform a stress test because they released me. After being released from the hospital, I followed up with Dr. Basco three days later.

At my visit, he asked if my symptoms had subsided or gotten worse. I looked at him and smiled and said, " now, Dr. Basco, you know nothing has changed other than my chest pain seems to have gotten a little worse, and I have more often. And to be honest, I'm so over it. His staff checked my blood, heart rate and did another EKG. When LaRhonda, his Nurse, came in the room and gave him my paperwork, he frowned.
He asked, " Charnique, has anyone ever her of WPW syndrome.
 I frowned " no. " What is it?
He said it's an uncommon type of heart disease that makes you feel like your heart race abnormally fast for 10 to 15 minutes, if not longer. Many people have ever heard that WPW's caused by an extra electrical connection in the heart you were born with, although it doesn't present itself until later in life. Dr. Basco went on to say that only 1 in 100,000 people are diagnosed annually due to a lack of research. I had to wait for almost two weeks for my appointment. He

wanted me to wear a heart monitor for 10 to 14 days to see if it captured any abnormalities. He did say that WPW was and is very hard to diagnose because capturing it was almost impossible.

The morning I was scheduled to have the Transesophageal Echocardiogram (TEE) and heart catheterization, my doorbell rang around 4:30. Only God knows how happy I was to see my Mom's face. She and my mother-in-law would be there when they rolled me back and when I came out. I was happy.

Finally, I was able to take a deep breath. After going over my family medical history, immediate and extended family, it turns out that I inherited some of my Father's heart problems. I didn't know my Dad was also born with a heart murmur and several other heart-related issues. Either way, I had to deal with it now.

Dr. Basco spoke instead of Tiana this time. He told me that he had some bad news and good news, and it was up to me to say to him which I wanted to hear first. I've always gone with the bad news first, so I told him to shoot for the stars. I'm all ears.

He started by telling me to try and stay calm as he explained.

The correct terms for what I have are mitral valve insufficiency, prolapse, tachycardia, cardiomyopathy, atrial fibrillation, edema, shortness of breath, and WPW. Everything he said sounded like french.

My mitral valve's primary concern was leaking so bad I had to get it repaired or replaced soon, or I wouldn't make it much longer. Dr. Basco sat down and scooted his chair closer before saying if I didn't have surgery, I might not live to see the age 35. In a nutshell, I need to have my mitral valve replaced or repaired as soon as possible. Dr. Basco thought my tricuspid valve was leaking at that time, but it was minor at a three, nothing of any significance. Everything was moving so fast for me. Dr. Basco's office referred me to see Dr. Joel Gooch, who was supposed to be one of the best heart surgeons in Memphis. He worked with Baptist East Memorial Hospital that following Tuesday at 9:00 that morning. My nerves and anxiety were all over the place. The office staff was so welcoming, and the wait time wasn't wrong either after sitting in the waiting room for less than 20 minutes before they called me back.

During my consultation, Dr. Gooch's bedside manner was excellent. He answered all of my questions and tried to make me feel confident in allowing him to crack my chest open and try to fix my valve.

Before my appointment, DeWayne and I sat down and made a list of all the questions he and I had regarding the day of surgery, recovery, and after.

My first question was:

1. How long does a typical open-heart surgery last?
2. How long would I be in ICU?
3. And how long would I be in the hospital after going to a regular room before being discharged?
4. What should I expect to see and feel when I wake up from all of the sedation medication?
5. How long would his office follow me after I'm released?

He and his office staff gave me all of the information I needed to go over before making a final decision. I rescheduled my follow-up appointment for Friday morning because I didn't want to waste any time talking myself out of saving my own life. When I got into the car, I sat there and cried. A million questions were going through my head at one time.

Why in the hell is this happening to me? Could I have done something to cause my heart problems, or was I born with all of this?

I put my dark shades on and drove home. I couldn't get my words together when I called Dewayne, so I opted to call him back when I made it home and got myself together. By the time I made it home, I was a wreck. I went inside and fell on the couch. I did have enough sense to call Dr. Gooch to speak with Keith, his lead Nurse. I needed something for my nerves if I would make the next two weeks for the open slot. Luckily, they agreed to call me something Xanax in to get me through, contingent on me keeping my appointment for Friday. Before hanging up, I told Keith, my husband and I were going out of town for my last hoorah at Six Flags theme park the weekend before my surgery. He laughed. I promised to keep my appointment, and we hung up.

I'd only been with Excellerx for a little over a year right before I had my first surgery. I wasn't sure if they'd let me go or try to work with being on leave of absence for 12 weeks. I knew that laws protect employees, but the bottom line is they have to make sure the business is making money and profitable.

Luckily, my team pharmacist supervisor Kirk was real laid back and willing to work with his team. Once my nerves settled, I spoke to him, and as expected, he told me to do what was best for me and keep him in the loop. He processed my paperwork with a tentative date of June 26, and tears started falling again. I was grateful.

Dewayne took three days off work the next day to be with me at my next follow-up appointment. I was shocked when he had some questions of his own.

My heart surgery was scheduled for June 26, 2006, at 6:00 that morning.

As requested, I'd be Dr. Gooch's first case. DeWayne and I left out around 4:30 Friday morning. I had a plan to enjoy myself before

I had surgery because I'd be missing the entire summer.

We had the entire weekend to shop, eat, drink, and do whatever else we could think of doing. We had a blast.DeWayne had taken his time and picked out one of the best hotels in St. Louis with a hot tub and some fantastic amenities that were to die for, and I loved it. Any other day I'd be somewhere trying to count calories and carbs, but not that weekend. I just needed to feel free. Free of everything. Dewayne and I made sure my last night of drinking for a minute was a good one that Saturday night. We walked down the strip to one of the local bar Wet Willey's, downtown, until almost 3:00 in the morning.

I drank everything from Patron shots to walk me downs, and I felt great. That was until my heart started pounding halfway back to our room. It was so intense I had to stop and almost lay on the ground before it eased up. The pain started in my chest and radiated from my neck down my arms. I scared the shit out of Dewayne. He was ready to take me to the hospital and have me admitted for the weekend. It took a minute, but I was able to talk him down. All we had to do was wait for Monday, and hopefully, all of my pain and worries would be behind us. I had to keep promising him I'd be okay. We left St. Louis midafternoon Sunday, hoping to beat some of the after-church Sunday crowd. When we made it home, I was surprised to see my mother-in-law at our house and cooking Sunday dinner. She'd cooked all of my favorites from fried chicken, scalloped potatoes, steamed broccoli, and yeast rolls. I almost cried, standing in the doorway of the kitchen. I didn't understand why I had to go through this.

I walked over to where she was standing and thanked her for giving me some normalcy and peace of mind. She had no idea what that moment meant to me, especially since I couldn't have anything to eat or drink after midnight that night. I ate and ate until I couldn't eat anymore.

The morning of my surgery, my nerves were everywhere, and my mind was everywhere and nowhere at the same time. I couldn't focus on anything. I called and talked to my Dad the night before, and I promised to call him before they rolled me back for surgery. My Dad had to know that just hearing his voice calling my name "Baby Girl," my worries left. I was ready for anything that came my way. I know what you're thinking. No, my Dad did not come to the hospital while I had surgery because he hates them. He promised to have someone drop him after I came out of ICU, which was good enough for me. I didn't want him to see me like that, nor did he. With all of the formalities out the way, I was ready. My Mom and my sister made sure I had enough pajamas, towels, undershirts, and most importantly, watermelon to get me through at least the first few weeks of post-op.

My family and I all piled in the pre-op area waiting room at Baptist East, making all kinds of small talk. At the same time, we waited in pre-op for them to call me back. I was surprised to see Kena and her boys show up. She told me she would be there, but I sometimes know people say things without any intentions of actually showing up. I think I must've been smiling from ear to ear when I come through the double doors. We didn't get a chance to talk that much before they called for only one guest and me at that time. The surgical team explained that everyone would get a chance to see me after getting all of my vitals, blood work, and IVs put in. It took about thirty minutes from start to finish for them to get me ready to roll back to surgery. Everybody came in to give their good wishes and promises to be there when I came out of recovery. Kena was the only person who wouldn't be there when I came out of surgery, but she promised to go in the next few days when I was out of the ICU or home.

 After just about everybody left the room except for Dewayne, Kena and her boys stood around me holding hands and began to pray for me to have a successful surgery and recovery. When Kena stopped praying, Bubba started, and before they could say amen, tears were rolling down my face and Kena's. Just as she and her boys left, the surgeon came back in to moved me around. My heart dropped. The brave face I'd been wearing was to give everyone else a piece of mind and replaced it with fear. Dewayne must have sensed my apprehension because he started holding on to my hands even tighter and whispering, "I was going to be okay," in my ear. Right then, I realized how much I loved this man. They allowed us to kiss one last time before I disappeared behind the surgical doors.

When I made it to my surgical room, Keith and the anesthesiologist were already waiting for me and smiling. They both repeated good morning and asked if I needed anything right then for my nerves. I almost cursed.

Yes, I do.

Once they transferred me to the surgical bed, Dr. Elise Parker was the anesthesiologist. She was ready for me; she had Benadryl and Lorazepam already drawn up in the syringe waiting for me. Feeling the lights shine against my skin only made my nerves worse than they already were. After that, the last thing I remember was seeing Dr. Gooch walked into the room, saying good morning and rubbing my arm.

Before Dr. Gooch could get his gloves on all the way, I said, "alright, I need you to remember I'm only 26 years old and I love showing off my breast. Please do not start my incision and the top of my collar bone". "Make sure it's a pretty scar that you can barely see." The entire surgical team started laughing.

That cleared the tension from the room. Elise pushed that Lorazepam and Benadryl. I felt like I was floating on a cloud without a care in the world.

The surgical team asked who my favorite artist was. How could I not say "India Arie" and her song? My favorite song, Video blasted on the overhead radio system within seconds?

I could hear "I'm not your average girl from your video" then "Beautiful Surprise."
Oh yeah.
Yall laughing, but I'm dead serious. I'll be stalking Dr. Gooch in the dark with a flashlight. Elise was still laughing. She said, okay ", I'm about to push the Propofol," and I need you to count to ten for me as she placed the oxygen mask over my nose and mouth. My world went black after that. When I woke up in recovery, the only face I saw was Dewayne sitting in the corner and a chair that looked pretty uncomfortable, and that was enough for me. He must've seen my eyes open because I could hear him calling for a nurse to come into the room. My heart was beating so fast and hard. The pain was unlike anything I had ever endured.
The nurses cleared out of the room, Dewayne came over to the bed, and those green eyes of his put my spirit at ease. I don't remember being in much pain the entire time I was in ICU, but it was a different beast when I made it to the Step-

Down Cardiac Unit. When I woke in the step-down Cardiac Unit, I still had tubes running everywhere in my neck, arms, and stomach, and I'd be lying. I said it didn't scare the hell out of me. The only thing they'd taken out so far was the intubation tube from my throat. That was way too much for me; I needed something for my nerves. I hit the call button twice so the Nurse could hopefully catch Keith or Dr. Gooch before they left the floor.

Dr. Gooch and his staff arrived early the following day to check on my sutures and incisions, Thursday, day four. He finally gave the okay for Keith to remove the breathing tubes from my abdomen. It hurt like hell.

I hadn't seen my incision, but they said it was looking great, and it was looking like I only had to stay in the hospital a few more days but not until I had a bowel movement. When the surgical team left the room, my nursing staff came in. Nurse Emily was holding a red pillow shaped like a heart that I'd need to use. They explained that anytime I made any movements such as shifting, coughing, or grunting, but no matter small, I needed to place the pillow to my chest firmly so my sternum would not move. They explained that I now had wires attached in three separate places holding my sternum in place so it could heal properly and fuse back together, and they would never come out.

Yeah, right, Dr. Gooch, for that to happen, I'd need a stool softener or a laxative and more than one.

Dr. Gooch started making small talk about the weather, and I was looking to take walks in the park and downtown on the river as he checked on the IVs in my neck. The surgical team and nurses were on their way out of my room when I asked them if they could remove the catheter because it was uncomfortable and starting to hurt. If I could've jumped out of bed when he said "yes," I would have. I felt like I was on a roll. I told Dr. Gooch my 26th birthday was in two weeks, and I wanted to be in my bed with my pretty tiny incision.

He turned back around and said, "trust me, Charnique, trust me with his perfect smile and his Botox-filled face.

 I was so over getting woken up at 2:00, 5:00 each morning when I'd just closed my eyes for blood work.

Day 5: Dr. Basco popped up around 4:30 in the morning, just as I was about to close my eyes. He had too much damn energy for 4:30 in the morning.

But just like any other time, I see him as he enters the room and says, "good morning Charnique, how are you feeling today"?

His bedside manner is always pleasant, and unlike most doctors I've seen, he has been straightforward with me no matter what. Speaking loud enough for my husband to hear what he said after your last set of lab work comes back, depending on the results, I think I don't have a problem discharging you. I thought my husband was asleep in the corner on the couch, but his head popped up then. He said, "don't listen to her. You all keep her as long as you need to.

Ugh, no.
I'm ready to get out of here. My labs came back about two later hours. So did the bad news. My Potassium, magnesium, and sodium levels had dropped because my Furosemide dose was so high temporarily, they hoped. I had to stay at least another day, and Lord knows I was praying for it to be just one more day.
Like clockwork, the lab came back in at 8:00 that night and again around 4:30 to 5:00 the following day.
My lab work finally came back, and I was good to go.
Yes.

At 12:30, the nursing staff was preparing my discharge paperwork.
I couldn't wait to call my Dad with my good news.
My grandmother answered on the third ring. She talked long enough for her to tell me my Dad had not slept or eaten in almost a week ago.

She yelled his name from the living room," Percy, come to the phone.
It's your Babygirl".
She sounds tired, so hurry up. I could hear my Dad laughing in this distance when he asked her if she was sure it was me.
Granny said," don't you think by now I'd know they know the difference in my grandchildren's voices by now." That child is almost 30. She's got jokes acting like I can't hear.
When I heard my Dad's voice coming through that phone, tears ran down my face.
He said, "Babygirl, Babygirl is that you"?
Through my tears, I said, "yes, Daddy, it's me."
My Dad has always talked faster and even faster when he gets excited.
So, everything is fine. When are you going home?
Hold on, Daddy, I'm going home today in a couple of hours at most. I could tell how happy he was in his voice.

Daddy, Granny said, you haven't slept in almost a whole week.

Is that true?

He tried to change the subject, but I knew him too well. He started stuttering, BabyGirl, and I couldn't rest until I knew you were okay and out of harm's way. I hope you can get some sleep ow since you've heard my voice.

It was time to go home. But, before the attendant could roll me out of the room, Nurse Emily stopped us and gave me another dose of Morphine just in case we had a long wait filling my prescriptions. They made my day. I couldn't wait for the sun to shine down on my skin. When the orderly rolled me outside where the patient's pickup was, I must've had the biggest smile on my face. It was something about the way summertime smelled and felt against my skin. It didn't help that I'm a July baby. It had to be about 90 degrees or higher, and for the first time, I had no complaints. Everybody piled in their vehicles and followed us back to our townhouse. Child, Memphis potholes were the absolute worse. I felt each and everyone we hit. The pain was horrible; I could only imagine how much worse it would have been if I hadn't just Morphine. When DeWayne opened the door, I smelled nothing but food. It was what I'd been missing this entire week. It was different from what I'd been smelling for the past week. I asked DeWayne who was cooking it was my mother-in-law, of course. Gail came flying through with Trotter right before her. Dewayne almost dropped everything in his hands, trying to catch her. She was coming straight for me at full speed. Making our way to the dining room, I could see a table full of food the closer we got. Gail had prepared everything chicken wings, macaroni, mashed potatoes, cabbage, cornbread, and chicken and dumplings just if I couldn't tolerate food yet. DeWayne and my younger brother Perry carried me upstairs to get me more comfortable before bringing a plate up. After everyone had eaten, they checked on me one last and made sure I had everything I needed before leaving out. Just like I'd asked Dewybne, he made sure to get me a mini-fridge so I wouldn't have to bug him or try to sneak downstairs by myself when he returned to work. My Mommy and oldest sister Yas made sure they hooked me up. They'd gotten grapes, oranges, apples, watermelon, and Captain Crunch, the peanut butter kind. Omg, they hooked me up. Everything after me trying to finish my food is a blur. I'm not sure how long I slept that day, but when that Morphine wore off, I almost lost my mind. Luckily, DeWayne had already gotten both my pain meds filled, and he came rushing up the steps when he heard me moving around in bed. Right then, I would have paid a million bucks for a Percocet if I had to. It took less than thirty minutes for it to kick in. I promise if I could help it, I would make sure to take them around the clock as prescribed, at least until I learn how to control the pain.

The first weeks went by like a blur with either me sleeping or trying to find something on TV to watch. One day, in particular, it must have been during week four or five. I was home alone, and Trotter would not stop whining and barking up a storm. My silly butt had gotten tired of feeling lonely, so I walked my butt down the steps, let her out of the kennel, and took her upstairs with me. Surprisingly, after we both gotten settled in the bed, she went straight to sleep.

I guess all she wanted was to be upstairs up under me. That was her way of protecting me. It was sweet. The kicker was I had to make it back down the steps before DeWayne made it back home, which didn't happen because he came home early. And Trotter snitched by running down the steps to greet him when she heard the car pull into the driveway. When he came upstairs, he said, so I see you've been busy.

I smirked and tried to avoid the question, but he didn't have it. He fussed and made me promise not to go back down the steps without him until I'd gotten a little bit stronger. If I agreed, he leaves Trotter out for me. After he'd gotten me settled back in bed temporarily as he brought some groceries he'd picked up for me. DeWayne had gotten me a few sour pickles, carrots, pretzels, chips, and a veggie tray. He made sure I didn't have to leave our bedroom unless I had to use the bathroom. After he had my attention with the snacks, he brought in the most hated object for any woman, a scale and a blood pressure machine. He said that we had to keep a record to follow the doctor's orders over the next two weeks.

I told him, "you know I would have been fine with a fridge full of watermelon and pickles."

I went from eating pickles the way they came in the bag to putting my sour pickle in a zip lock bag and adding salt and hot sauce. I'm not sure why but I craved salt. After doing my research, I learned the body craves what was being depleted by my fluid pills. I went from buying pickles in the store to learning how to pickle cucumbers on my own.

DeWayne asked me what time my next appointment was on Thursday as he was walking down the steps. I yelled down the hall. It's at 10:15. He said, good and kept down the stairs with his arms full.

Thursday morning had come fast, it was time for my six-week checkup with Dr. Gooch, and I was ready to have some of my restrictions lifted. It was my first time having any surgery. I had no idea about what to expect. When we arrived fifteen minutes before my appointment, the office staff was sent straight back to one of the examination rooms.

I looked over at DeWayne. No wait time, that's new.

Dr. Gooch and his Nurse Julianne came in minutes later, and just like any other time, he was wearing his million-dollar smile.

He said, Charnique, how have you been? Any concerns, any changes?

Nothing that I can think of other than when my pain will get better?

Well, Charnique, it's hard to say because it differs from patient to patient. So, for patients, it takes a few weeks, others it months, even years.

Why don't you show me where the pain is and tell me a little about what you are doing when you experience pain the most? I pointed to my sternal region and the area right below and explained it was when I raised my arms or reached anything, no matter how far or close. And that the pain gets worse and radiates across my chest the worse. At the same time, Dr. Gooch explained that it would require time and for me to have a lot of patience while I tried to get back to where I was before. Keith tried to slide into the examination room quietly behind Dr. Gooch. Dr. Gooch told Julianne that he would increase my Lortab to 10mg/650 every 6 to 8 hours and keep me on Percocet 5/325 every 4 to 6 hours as needed. Keith slid over to where I was sitting and asked to open the gown so Dr. Gooch could hopefully remove the tape covering my incision and look at the stitches. I was so afraid to look at my incision, DeWayne scooted closer and held my hand as he pulled the tap off. After taking a good look at it, Keith handed me a mirror. I would be lying if I said I wasn't shocked. It looked great, and a lot of the swelling had already started going down. The only problem Dr. Gooch saw was a few of my stitches hadn't started dissolving or become loose enough for removal. Dr. Gooch instructed Keith or Julianne to replace it with a different kind for sensitive skin, and hopefully, it would allow my skin to breathe more. He'd leave it on for another three or four weeks just to be safe.

After leaving my appointment, DeWayne took me out to one of my favorite restaurants before taking me home from Chili's Rresuraunt. I ordered my usual appetizers, buffalo wings, loaded fries, and for my entrée, the chicken and shrimp fajitas. Even though my appetite had changed for the worse, I stuck with my tradition. If I couldn't eat all of it, I would hopefully take it home to finish later that night. When we left there, I felt like a million bucks, and our next stop was Walgreens to get my new prescriptions filled. I was glad to see a familiar face working the drop-off window, which only meant my wait time would not be longer than 15 to 20 minutes. So we browsed the store until Shameeka called my name for me to pick up my medicine from the pharmacy. So we were walking around the store about to spend money we needed to be saving because I was only getting 60 percent of my check.

Over the next few weeks, DeWayne started trying to get back into our routine. We started trying to take short walks, to begin with adding on another block each week. Even though Dr. Gooch and Dr. Basco told me they doubted that I'd ever been able to go running again. Anyone that knows me knows that I hate restrictions, but most importantly, I hate for someone to tell me what I can do or they think I'd do again. I insisted on proving them wrong. Even though I knew it was dangerous, I couldn't sit still and do anything. I had to take charge.

When I was sure my husband had pulled out the driveway, I'd call My dog Trotter upstairs, put her leash on her and slip on some tennis shoes.

Within three weeks, one block turned into two, two turned into three, and four turned into me walking a mile or two with no problem. After that, I pushed myself to jog a block until I could run without any issues.

Five months rolled around before I knew it, and all of my symptoms came right along with the six months. I found myself back in Dr. Basco complaining about chest pain, dizziness, shortness of breath, and how debilitating it had become. We tried switching up my meds for about two weeks, but that didn't help. My next step after that was another set of tests. I had to have another TEE's, Echo's, stress test, and heart catheterization done. Dr. Basco put the orders in as stat to have my results back within no more than two days. Dewayne

couldn't take off work, but luckily my Mom and Mother-in-Law Gail could be there with me to drive me home. I was on edge, waiting for those results. I couldn't eat or sleep. When I got the phone call around 1:00 Wednesday afternoon, nothing could have prepared me for it. I was at work. Dr. Basco said, Charnique, are you somewhere you can sit down and talk for a minute. The tone of his voice was enough to have tears rushing down my cheeks.
I placed my phone on break and walked away from my desk. I walked outside, hoping to find somewhere to sit down away from everybody else without going to my car. After sitting down, I said, okay, tell me what's going on.
He said, "it's not looking good. Your mitral valve is leaking worse than it was before." I need you to hang with me and call Dr. Gooch's office for an appointment if that's possible, or would you like for my office to make your appointment and call you back. For a moment, I was speechless. I'd done everything that was required. My diet

wasn't bad, and I exercised three to four times a week already.
What did I do wrong?
I was confused.
I said, "okay." Give me one second to process this. I took a deep breath and told him to have one of his nurses call for the first available appointment and give me a callback.
Right then, the only thing I could think of was I knew something was wrong. I could only walk more than six to seven feet without having to stop and sit down. Dr. Basco said I'm just happy one came into the office as soon as you did. I thanked him for listening to me as I walked back into the office, on my way down the hall to see Kirk, my supervisor. I told him what was happening and that I needed to leave for the day.
He said, of course, call me if you need anything. I filled my Kena, Stephanie, and Sandra in as I closed out my computer and headed for the door. Instead of calling my Mom first, I called DeWayne. I knew he was

just as worried as me. He answered on the second ring, asking if okay.

No, not really, but are you free to talk for a minute. I explained what was going on and that I'd left work for the day. He told me I shouldn't be alone right, so he was about to call dispatch to take off for the rest of the day and meet me home. DeWayne made it home fifteen to twenty minutes after I did. His green eyes were brown, and I could see the hurt on his face. He reached out for me as soon as he made it through the front door. All that I could do was fall into his arms with tears running down my face. He tried his best to calm me. He kept repeated I got you. I need you to calm down so you don't make yourself sick, so you don't start having chest pain. We don't need that right now. Just know Dr. Basco listened to you; hopefully, we caught it in time. Unfortunately, it was already too late for that. The stress was too much. DeWayne ended calling an ambulance. When they arrived, the first thing they tried was Nitroglycerin and Aspirin. Without thinking

about I took Nitroglycerin. That damn thing could have killed me. It wasn't until DeWayne heard the EMT ask if it was helping any. I'd forgotten to tell DeWayne and my Mom about my appointment on Monday morning at 8:15.
I shook my head "no."
DeWayne slammed his hand against the ambulance door and said, "damn it, she's not supposed to take Nitroglycerin. She has WPW." The EMT's eyes got big as hell. By then, I couldn't speak. The pain had gotten worse.
As usual, I knew they'd run a whole lot of tests, including an EKG, when I made it to the hospital, and I couldn't stand it. Because no matter what was happening to me, nothing showed up except when there was an episode of WPW occurring right then. The EMT got the driver's attention and told him they needed to turn on the lights. They needed to get me to Methodist North Hospital without me coding. The EMT gave me a dose of adrenaline, hoping to speed up my heart rate, even if it was just for a

few minutes. We pulled up to the hospital in what felt like a matter of minutes. After checking me in, they put me in a room and immediately started pushing fluids and hooking me up to my most-hated machine, the EKG. The ER doctor came into the examination room and told me that they needed to keep me at a minimum overnight. I wasn't surprised, but I gave them Dr. Basco and Dr. Gooch's phone numbers so he could consult with them and hopefully understand my heart problems. They wanted to run more tests. I waited for almost an hour for the ER to call Dr. Basco. When the doctor finally came back into the room, he stated that he and Dr.Basco agreed on allowing this round of fluids to continue, then discharging you with strict instructions to keep your appointment with your heart surgeon.

I looked up at him, thanked him, and told him keeping my appointment was something he didn't have to worry about. The ER nurse came in two hours later with a lot of information regarding WPW and

Atrial Fibrillation, along with my discharge papers. She explained what could happen if one of my episodes became too severe, leading to death.

When she left out the door, I told Dewayne Dr. Basco called back earlier, and my appointment was for April 9, 2007, at 8:15. I thanked her and promised to go over the do's and don't first thing in the morning. When we made it back home, it was almost midnight. There was no way in the world I could make it to work the next day without possibly passing at my desk. After calling my job and leaving Kirk a voicemail, I passed out in bed.

The following day around 11:00, my phone rang. Looking at the caller ID, it was Dr. Basco's office. The first thing I could think of was, "what could it possibly be now." But shockingly, it was Dr. Basco just trying to see how I was doing and if my symptoms had come back.

I told him about the on-again and off-again chest pain radiating pain across my chest from time to time.

Dr. Basco told me to "try to alleviate stress if at all possible." He knew it would be challenging given the circumstances, but it may also help me with my second surgery, along with me being patient.

Fighting my tears back, I told him I'd try and thanked him for checking up on me. It meant a whole lot to me.

March was already over, and April was flying by. I was hoping to go out of town to shop and get some stuff to enjoy the weather, but that would not happen. It was an hour before my appointment time, and I was freaking out. I was a little disappointed that Dewayne and my Mom couldn't take off, but I was able to get my Mother-in-inlaw, Gail, to go along with me. As usual, I only had to sit in the room for about ten minutes before Keith called me to the back examination rooms. I was on edge. A few minutes later, Dr. Gooch came into the room holding my latest results.

Charnique, why are you back so soon?

I looked at him and said, "really, Dr. Joel Gooch, tell me where I'm looking at."

Dr. Gooch said, "I assume Dr. Basco has already told you that repair didn't work and that your Mitral Valve is leaking worse than before.

I couldn't get a word out, but I shook my head "yes" in agreement.

He explained this time, and I needed to have my valve replaced. And with this surgery, I had four options that were available at that time. A biological heart valve was a pig valve, mechanical valve, bioprosthetic, and donor valve. Without much thinking, I agreed to the bioprosthetic through St.Jude. Because it was the safest, and it meant I didn't have to take Warfarin for the rest of my life.

Dr. Gooch explained that he would have to crack my chest open, making the odds more challenging to predict.

But he and his team would be doing their best to make sure that I was stable and doing great when they walked out of that operating room. Keith stepped out of the room long enough to grab the calendar with the surgery dates available. Of course, I had to pick a Monday morning, but I had to be his patient, so I went with April 23, 2007, at 6:00 am. I was his first patient that morning which was what I wanted.

It was something about never wanting a surgeon that's been on duty for 36 hours straight that scared the shit out of me. I knew too much about how many doctors and surgeons end up losing them or making major mistakes and killing their patients.

I chose the date and handed Keith the folder back. Dr. Gooch gave me before he let me he needed to take a look at my sternum and breastbone. That only took about five minutes, and after that, we were headed back to the car.

I called DeWayne on my way back home to make sure he had enough time to request off my surgery. He asked if I was sure I could make two weeks.

I felt like I could, and that gave us enough time to everything in order. After hanging up with DeWayne, I called my Mom and sister Yas three-way, so I wouldn't have to repeat anything. My Mom had no problem

taking off, and she had enough sick and vacation banked to be off for at least three months if she ever needed it. Yas told me that Mosque 55 had a fish fry to raise money for the school, and she'd already volunteered to help with the cooking.
I can't lie.
Why wouldn't my siblings be there for me? Anytime they'd needed me, I'd always be there for her no matter what?
I took a deep, and I sucked it up and asked if the school would be open on April 20 so I could bring Zoe's birthday presents, cake, and ice cream.
It was the weekend before my surgery. I'd gotten up early enough to pick up Zoe's cake and deliver it to the school. And I'd made plans for DeWayne and me to go to the movies, out to eat at Owen Brennan's, and to go downtown on Beale later that evening. I was dressed up, drunk, and ready to go out and have fun. I'd taken five or six shots of Patron, and I was stuffed from dinner and by 10:30. I was far more exhausted and regretting drinking those

shots faster than I usually would. I slept just about all Sunday, and I got out the bed long enough to eat lunch and dinner. I still couldn't believe that I'd had my first heart surgery in June of last year, and now I'm back at square A having to relive the pain and agony all over again. Later that night, when I got back up, I looked over to the clock ad noticed I still had almost two hours before I had to cut off food and liquids until after my surgery. I jumped out of bed and ran down the steps to find food. I didn't want anything heavy. I just needed a snack. I grabbed the Doritos from the cabinets, a Sprite, Whooper candies, and a pickle. I would be complete or almost total this time instead of starving for 12 to 14 hours or longer.

It was 3:00 in the morning on April 23, and time for me to get up. I had to take another shower, wipe down with the special disinfecting wipes, put the Bactroban ointment inside of each nostril, dress, and more than anything, I had to make sure I was in a positive mental space.

Time was flying, it was already 4:15, and I had to be at the hospital and checked in no later than 4:45. I'm guessing everybody noticed that time at the same time and started heading for the car. When we made it to the Baptist East, I felt like I would throw up all over myself. This time my support team included everybody except both of my sisters. My oldest sister had a separate engagement that she didn't want to miss, and my other sister was still in prison for something I wouldn't talk about. I did have my husband DeWayne, my mother, brother, and some extended family. I had enough support there that allowed me to feel loved, and it gave me the strength and courage to face the obstacle in front of me.

At 5:00 am, the surgical team came to the door and called my name to go to pre-op. It took them forever to get the IV started. By the time they finished, I had looked like a walking pin cushion. I was in the same position I was before. It was almost time for me to roll back to the operating room. I kissed my family and held on to DeWayne as long as I could. Once, I heard my husband yell, I love you down the hall, and my heart was at ease. The nerves went away.

It was once again time. Dr. Elise was there with my cocktail waiting as I wheeled into the surgical suite. She spoke and held up the syringe smiling from ear to ear.
She said I got you, Charnique.
I burst out laughing.
They transferred me to the surgical bed. I closed my eyes and said a silent prayer. When I opened my eyes, I told Dr. Elsise to go ahead and give me something for my nerves. Dr.Gooch came into the room with tons of energy, as I expected. He was wired and ready to go.
 Dr. Gooch came closer to me and asked if I was comfortable and ready to start while putting on his surgical gown and gloves.
Dr. Gooch "yes," the readiest I would ever be.
The last thing I remember is hearing him telling the team, let's get the show on the

road and Dr. Elise telling me to count backward to ten.

I'm not sure how long my surgery took, but I remember smelling DeWayne's cologne as I tried to open my eyes. I was looking forward to rolling back into a room and knowing he was there.

Dewayne has always been one of my favorite colognes, so I would know he was there no matter what.

I could feel the intubation tube still down my throat and wires going in and out of my body when coming out of sedation. I tried not to freak out, but I couldn't help it. It was freaking out. I finally opened my eyes, and the first person I saw was Dewayne sitting right by my side. He kept saying, "baby, it's okay try to calm down, or they're going to give you a sedative." But it was hurting so bad. I felt like my throat was literally on fire. I needed it out, and now. I reached up once again. This time I felt someone pull the intubation out of my throat with a sense of urgency. Even though I was on a lot of pain meds, I knew something wasn't right.

I was fully awake a day or so after my surgery. I felt fine, but as always, I had a ton of questions. One would be how long my surgery was?

And were there any complications? According to my family, they said it lasted almost eight and ½ hours from start to finish. At one point, they'd gotten an update from Dr.Gooch at the midway point explaining that I'd lost a lot of blood and obtained authorization to start a blood transfusion. Just as the words left his mouth, I looked over to my right at my IV pole, and there was another bag hanging behind it.

I felt tears threatening to roll down my face. I looked back over to where DeWayne was sitting and asked if there was anything else. He replied, "nope."

I laid my head back and thanked the "Most High." I'd made it once again. Tears flooded my face.

DeWayne rushed over to the bed and grabbed my hand.

Niki, I need you to hear me and look in my eyes. You were touch and go for the last two days, but you made it through. You are okay, and you made it through. There aren't many people that can go under the knife twice within nine months, but you did it, and you will be walked over around this unit at some point today. Be grateful and live in this moment. He told me, "I love you." I have your back. No worries, okay. Damn, I love this man. I could only imagine what I looked like, but he loved me anyway.

Why?

Would he eventually regret being by my side?

How can he possibly put my mind at ease so quickly?

Taking a deep, I let it all go. I'd made it through the most challenging part. The only thing that was left was me doing my part to strengthen my heart.

I remember waking up with my Nurse, and Nurse Sandra stand over me, trying to take my temperature without waking me up. When she noticed I was awake, she said, "there you are" I've been waiting for you to wake up.

How are you feeling?

As bad as I wanted to tell her I was in a lot of pain, I couldn't. My throat was dry so that I couldn't say much. When she noticed the grimacing look on my face, she offered me a sip of water and a couple of ice chips. It took me a second before I could speak because my throat was still raw. It took me a minute, but I managed to tell I felt overall, but my pain level was about a ten and ½ out of 10. I didn't have to say much else. My world went black. The next time I remember being awake, I was in the stepdown unit on day 4. I knew things weren't going to be as easy as it was for me his time because they were opening an incision that was just starting to heal, and my sternum was just being too fuse. Dr. Gooch explained that I would hurt a little more, but it didn't prepare me for this type of pain. The pain was excruciating. It was different in more ways than one.

Even though it was my fourth day in, I wasn't allowed to get out the bed. Dr. Gooch left strict instructions to lay almost flat with slight elevation for my entire hospital stay.
When the nurses explained it to me, I was confused as hell.
Why?
Are you sure?
In unison, they said "yes," no exceptions.
Dr. Basco and Dr.Gooch made sure we all knew that you are in the medical field and you'd try to get your way.
Really.
I called both of their names and asked them where my heart pillow was?
The hospital couldn't find me one.
I had both of them looking everywhere for one heart pillow. Call me crazy if you want, but that thing works magic.
Day 4 was pretty much easygoing. That was until I looked up and saw Keith coming through the door. I knew from my last surgery my breathing tubes and the tubes in my neck needed to come out. Let me be

honest there is nothing like someone pulling a set of 17 gauge needles out of your neck or boxes as long as my forearm out of your stomach. Not to mention. They have the nerve to say try to relax and breathe. It'll be quick.
Uh, no.
 DeWayne stayed close to me to make sure I followed the doctor's orders the entire time. I did everything they told me so I could take my butt home.

     Days 5 and 6 went by fast; it was finally the morning of day 7. I was up at 5:30, waiting on the nursing to take their samples, temperature, and whatever else they could think. This time I didn't care at all. I even asked how long would it take for my labs to come back. I knew the drill. I couldn't go home until my labs, bloodwork, and vitals all had to be stable. It didn't take as long as I thought it would. By 12:30, both Dr. Gooch and a couple of his staff were walking in with smiles on their faces.
He and Keith reiterated that I would have to follow my instructions to the letters to

avoid any major setbacks. Keith adjusted my bed and told me to relax; he needed to take off the sterile tap and look at the incisions on my chest and legs. I forgot to mention while sedated, Dr. Baso also did a heart catheterization to ensure your doctor doesn't have any major mistakes. Typically most incisions are 2 or 3 inches long on the inner groin of either thigh, neck, or wrist with a wire about 0.9 diameters around. Neither one are any fun.

Once all of the wires, tubes, and the majority of the IVs come out, you start to feel a little better. I wasn't too sure; maybe I should call it apprehensive and fear. After all, I was only 26, about to be 27 years old. It was a lot to take in in a few weeks. Dr. Gooch gave me the best news I could have gotten that day. He'd already started my paperwork, and he wanted to tell me himself that I'd be going home today. Suppose I could have jumped from that hospital bed and ran down the hallway and out the door. I settled for the wheelchair.

I made it home safe and sound. Just like before, my mother-in-law was there cooking up a ton of food that I may not eat until later that night or the day after. Either way, I was grateful. My family made sure I was comfortable before heading out. The next few weeks went by like a blur; I spent most of it in bed, only getting up to shower and change into a different pair of pajamas. The was still so much pain. Anytime I moved my arms above shoulder level, it seemed like something popped or shifted more than not. I tried to look over and just that everything was fine.

Every morning when I'd wake up, there be a bluebird sitting on my air conditioner chirping up a storm at the time. He never missed a day. By week 7, I felt like my angel came to give me peace of mind and calm me down. Dewayne would leave every morning around 7:00, so I would call alone, just myself and Trotter. I knew that to start feeling like myself. I had to get out of bed and start moving around. By midweek, I'd started a new routine. I'd get up, change into some workout clothes, and hope to hear my little friend outside my windowsill. I gave it the Tito and watched for him every morning before I started my day.

 Most days, by 7:45, I was headed out the door to take a walk toward Rhodes College. I started slow, nothing too major. I started off walking one block. Eventually, that turned into me being able to walk five blocks. I was jogging from our townhouse up to North Parkway, then around Rhodes College and back. I was so proud of myself. That helped me drop all of the fluid weight and hospital weight I gained. When I saw the scale go from 186 back down to 169, you couldn't tell me anything. I felt like I was back.

I wish more doctors would talk to patients about depression, self-doubt, and apprehension about any signs like heart surgery. I knew something was going on with me, but I couldn't put my finger on it. DeWayne was spending more and more at work or with his friends, so that he couldn't help. I had to get through myself.

All of my checkups went great, and it was about time for me to start thinking about going back to work. But one morning after DeWayne had left for work, the HR department from work called. I thought they were calling to check on my recovery or see when I was returning to work. Unfortunately, the phone took a left turn. It went something like this.

"This is Michelle from Excellerx's HR department."
 Do you have a minute?
Of course, Charnique. You don't have to be so formal.
She says I know, but these phone calls are recorded.
My first thought was, ugh.
Michelle was calling because your 12 weeks are almost up, and I've been informed that we have to terminate your employment because you've already exhausted all of your FMLA time. She did have the authorization to offer me the third shift position with the same pay.

I asked, are you sure?

Michelle, there is no way to work that shift while I'm still trying to recover from heart surgery.

Do I have another option?

That was the only thing she could offer me at that time. I told her I'd give my decision within the next 48 hours.

I pondered and pondered over and over what I would do before calling DeWayne. He answered after the third ring. I hesitated. Try not to get upset, okay.

I just got off the phone with the HR department at my job. To make a long story short, she told me I was in jeopardy of losing my job.

DeWayne asked me, why?

I explained further. I'd already taken FMLA last April for my first heart surgery. I was out for 14 weeks, and some days I couldn't work after that. Now with this surgery, I've been out for ten weeks so far. They are terminating me but offering to rehire me if I work the 1:30 to 10:00 at night with the

same pay, but if I don't take, I lose my
benefits and insurance.
His response was, "hell no." Just like that.
Don't worry about it, we can go ahead and
get married and I'll you to my insurance
that way you'll be straight.
That's your idea of a proposal. I know we've
been planning it anyway. You are crazy.
I hoped he couldn't hear me crying, but I
was. There he was again, being my knight
and shining armor for me during what could
have become a nightmare for me.
That was my answer, and I am still waiting
for two days to call Michelle back. I wasn't
sure if my feelings were hurt or pissed off,
but I had to do what was best for me, and
at that point in my recovery, I couldn't risk
having a setback because I was rushing back
to work.
That was the first time I'd been without a
job since I started working in 1994, but it
was going to be okay. I had a lot going on
with me that I didn't understand, so I still
needed to take it slow. At my last visit with
Dr. Gooch, he explained I'd never been able

to go running again, and I'd have to take it slow until we were my body wasn't going to reject the bioprosthetic heart valve. He explained every patient is different, and there was no way of knowing this would be a good match, so I had to take it slow.

Ugh. If there's nothing in this world that I hate, I hate for anyone to tell me what I can or wouldn't be able to do.

There had to be a way for me to get back to some normalcy. Over the next week or two, I tried to push myself further. Instead of walking or jogging the neighborhood, I tried adding Taebo back into my routine just to get my cardio up a little bit. That was a terrible idea, and I think I did more harm than good. I'd have to stick with walking and jogging for a while.

The same day I called and told Michelle I declined her offer to work nights, I started looking for another job. It didn't take me long at all. I sent my resume to a few agencies, filled out countless applications, and had three interviews set up by Monday morning of the following week.

I was sending up all kinds of praises. I was
so afraid of not having my own money.
Don't ask me why. I knew throughout
everything DeWayne had my back, and he
would always provide no matter what. Most
people would never understand why but I'd
go under the knife a second time. I wasn't
raised to give up. A woman should always
have her own money, no matter what.
It was the most challenging surgery of the
two and more than I thought I'd ever go
through. There were so many days I'd sit in
my bedroom with the door closed crying.
My emotions were all over the place. I had
mixed feelings, one minute, I was happy as
hell, and the next, I'd be asking God why
me.

Why did I have to go through this again?
What could I have done to deserve all the
pain I'm going through?
Why did it have to hurt so bad?
The answer was simple, and nobody ever
said this life would be easy. If I keep on
living, there will be a lot of trials and

tribulations. I'd just have to learn to take life as it comes and not allow it to break me down.

It was months I'd had my second heart surgery but still had sutures along my incision that hadn't dissolved or fallen. I'm not fallen off. If I'm not mistaken, it was almost 18 months after surgery when I started pulling in the center of my chest, and it started oozing pus. Before making an appointment, I got a suture kit from work and removed the excess stitches myself. That didn't work out too well. I ended up right back in Dr. Gooch's office. My appointment went smoothly, and I only waited for about ten minutes before Keith called my name and led me to an exam room. Dr. Gooch came straight into the room, did his assessment, and returned with some Xylocaine and a suture kit a few minutes later. I'd be lying if I say it didn't hurt when he pulled those three stitches out.
Oh, my God.
Dang, it wasn't the words I chose bit it'll do.

It'd had been almost two years since my second surgery, and I was trying everything I could to get back to where I was physically before having my heart problems front and center. I started getting early in the morning before work or after work, either jogging to doing Taebo. I thought everything was going well. I'd even lost 15 pounds, and I was feeling good.

DeWayne planned a big trip for us that year to cruise to Mexico for six nights and five days. I needed that more than anything, and so did he. When I say he had my back, it would be an understatement. Anytime I moved the wrong or cried out for, he'd already been awake looking at me, trying to see what was wrong. It was amazing to see how careful and attentive he was with me. I had to learn how to move, sit up straight, and lean forward, but no one tells how painful it would be. Yes, the doctors give as many Percocet, Hydrocodone, Hydromorphone tablets as you would like but the meds numb your body and hinder your recovery. It's like a win-lose, which is better? Trust me, and I took Lortab for years due to my sternum continuing to when I moved. After completing surgery, my doctors and hospital staff no one mentioned rehab to me. I had to form a program and regimen with my heart and muscle strength. Either way, I was grateful to have made it through the second and came out on the other side of those operating rooms. The second heart surgery was challenging; I almost died. I carried the thought with me every day. At 27 years old, I almost died.

Almost three years to the day, I started having the same symptoms again. The chest pain was more intense, and my fluid retention was much worse than before. I'd started having rustling on the right side of my chest. At first, my PCP thought I had another viral infection or an upper respiratory infection, but I needed to make an appointment with my cardiologist to have an Echo done.

I felt that no matter what I did, the result was always going to be the same. I should've had a permanent chair in the waiting room with my name reserved for me.

I was tired of crying, tired of screaming, and tired of feeling as though my heart was going to give out on me no matter what I did. Monday morning at 8:15, I was sitting in traffic trying to make it to my 8:45 appointment with Dr. Basco with tears running down my face. Finally, making it five minutes early, I sat in the waiting room, waiting to hear my name. Just moments before Justin opened the door, I started having chest pains, and I felt like I was about to pass out. My feet felt so heavy I barely made it through the door. After taking my vitals, he looked up at me and asked, " if I was feeling okay"?

My skin felt clammy, and I was sick to my stomach.

The chest pain was so bad I couldn't speak, so I shook my head no. Before I could get a word out, Justin had already stepped into the hallway and called for help. Lucky for me, Dr. Basco's north office was directly behind Methodist North, but they called an ambulance to transport me instead of allowing me to drive just in case I had a heart attack. The ambulance got there in mere minutes. After loading in the ambulance, the EMT started an IV and pushed 1ml of epinephrine. Getting the IV started took longer than the ambulance ride. The Emergency room doctor assessed before ordering an EKG, chest X-ray, and an Echocardiogram STAT. It took a few hours but, as usual, they couldn't find anything wrong. After being discharged, Dr. Johnston gave me a prescription for Lortab to help with chest wall pain and Xanax to help with my anxiety. If nothing else pissed me off, blowing me off as though I didn't know what I was feeling, sure in the hell did. Over the next few days, il stayed home from work to rest before returning to work and hopefully before going back to Dr. Basco's office. I was able to get back in for an appointment on Friday afternoon.

Dr. Basco looked over my discharge paperwork, and he was just as confused as I was.

I'd had atrial fibrillation related to Wolff-Parkinson White Syndrome (WPW), causing the electrical wires in my heart to misfire. Dr. Basco scheduled me to have another Echo, Stress test, and heart cath on the following day, with my test beginning at 7:15. My emotions were all over the place. Would I die before I reached 35, as Dr. Basco said if I decided to do nothing?

What did I do to deserve this type of punishment?

Did my God hate me?

I was going through a different type of hell. I had undergone more procedures than anyone two to three times my age. I got a call early Thursday morning as I was on my way to work from Dr.Basco. He'd just finished reading my test results, and my tricuspid and mitral valve were leaking to the point where he'd say severely. His advice was to have heart surgery again to replace both as soon as possible. I stopped my car and pulled over to the side of the expressway to get myself together. Even though I knew I was wrong, I followed my first mind and made an appointment, but still, it hurt. I fought like hell to recovery, but it seemed like it was all for nothing. Dr. Basco had always been honest with me and straight to the point. I knew he could hear the pain in my voice when I tried to ask him questions. I needed to see if I would be a heart transplant candidate or was just supposed to continue having my chest cracked open every couple of years. Of course, there was no way for him to know for sure, but he did ensure that I didn't need a new heart, nor was I a candidate for one.

A third heart surgery.

Are you serious?

Would I make it through another surgery this soon?

I made an appointment to see Dr. Gooch two weeks later. This time my Rock made sure he was there with me. It took me forever to make it from the car to the elevator and the office. My wait in the waiting room and our time in the exam room were no more than thirty minutes tops. Dr. Gooch took longer looking over my records than he did talking.

Dr. Gooch stumbled over his words when he spoke, and he said, "Charnique, after carefully looking over your files, I don't think I'd be successful performing a successful, but I know a Cardiac Surgeon who would be." I looked him dead in his eyes, disappointed that he wouldn't be in the operating room with me because, at that point, I trusted him. He told a doctor that works at Vanderbilt Hospital located in Nashville trained him named Dr. Michael Petracek, and he was highly talented and excellent with complicated cases. To ease my fears, Dr. Gooch went on to say, once my date was set in stone, he'd travel with my family or meet us there. Before leaving, he had me stop at the front desk for the information I needed for Dr. Petracek.

First thing Monday morning, I was on the phone with Vanderbilt setting my first appointment. Dr. Petracek's in-office days were Friday's mostly, so I had to wait for three to get in for a visit. It was scheduled for August 14, 2009, at 9:00. There was nothing to prepare me for where I was at that moment.

I was beyond lost and confused; I was scared and afraid of what was about to happen to me. After jumping through hoops to get off work, it was finally time for us to get on the road to Nashville.

We waited for almost an hour for Dr. Petracek to come into my exam room. He came in and introduced himself before getting right to the point.

Dr. Petracek said, " I looked over your records with my Cardiac team, and the imagery that Dr. Basco and Dr. Gooch sent wasn't done with updated technology. If it is okay with you, I'd like my team to redo the TEE, stress test, heart catheterization, and maybe one to two more here.

Of course, if you feel your equipment will give you a better view of my heart. At that appointment alone, Dr. Petracek made me feel confident in him and his abilities. He was straightforward and honest with everything I asked.

Dr. Petracek said, "I need you to understand if I don't see severe leakage, I'd make an alternative plan. Before I could get a question out DeWayne, said, "thank you." We're not trying to rush her back under the knife unless it is necessary.

I was able to complete everything except the Stress test, which is the treadmill test. I think I walked for thirty seconds before having to sit down. I got a phone call from Dr. Petracek's Nurse two weeks later, and he felt my heart wasn't stronger enough to make it through surgery. He planned to increase my diuretics, change my diet.

After having what felt like my tenth TEE, my throat became more sensitive no matter what food or milk I tried to get down. When I tried to swallow food or liquids, my throat seemed to be on fire constantly. I tried dealing with it without going to an ENT, but it only got worse. After three months of straining to swallow, I eventually lost my voice.

When I say my plate was already full. I was ready to give up and throw in the towel. Dr. Petri was pleasant and very understanding of my situation. After placing an ultrasound tube down my nose and into my throat.

She diagnosed me with vocal cord fatigue, dysphagia, and a narrowing esophagus. But she couldn't tell me how long I'd be hoarse nor when I'd be able to swallow more than smoothies and Ensure.

At my previous appointment, Dr. Petracek mentioned I am trying the Atkins diet or Weight Watchers to help me lose about 30 pounds. Dewayne and I changed our diet entirely by eating clean. We fixed most of our meals at home, thoroughly cleaning our meat and vegetables and growing herbs and vegetables that we could in our backyard.

It still wasn't enough.

As time flew by fast and my heart got weaker and weaker. I'd gone from being able to walk three to four miles a day to not being able to walk ten steps without having to stop and sit down. My breathing got worse, and I had no idea why. At one of my visits, Dr. Petracek scheduled an appointment to have my Respiratory Specialist, which freaked me out. I had to put stuff over my head, in my mouth, and around my chest, then enter a booth. It was creepy. The Respiratory therapist didn't find any abnormalities that affected my lungs. Dr. Petracek and Dr. Byrd went back to the drawing board with the Cardiac team to find a reason for my symptoms and the cause of my severe heart disease. They knew it was hereditary, but it only explained the heart murmur because my Dad had no other problems. At my age, there was no explanation for WPW, cardiomyopathy, atrial fibrillation, congestive heart failure, Mitral prolapse and regurgitation, and Tricupside valve regurgitation. My cardiac team at Vanderbilt watched me closely. I had appointments set for every six to have either a TEE or Echocardiogram to monitor how well the walls of my heart were pumping. Even so, with doing all of that somewhere between June 2010 and May 2011, I had a mild attack that went unnoticed until I had TEE in June.

Why?

How could it be overlooked when I'm always in either Dr. Basco's office or Vanderbilt?

 Why is that out of all of my Mom's and Dad's children, did I have to be the one to be sick?

Dr, Petracek made me as comfortable as I could be for almost seven full years by overloading me with diuretics. At first, take Lasix 80mg twice daily, Spironolactone 5mg once a day, and Chlorothiazide 500mg once daily. Over time the Lasix stopped working, so he changed me to Torsemide 40mg twice daily, which worked well, but it still didn't pull everything off me.

A few months into 2014, my breathing became even more labored, and the chest pain was unbearable. Unlike most heart patients, I couldn't take Nitroglycerin for chest pain because I have WPW. It would kill me. I'm not sure what changed, but whatever it was, it changed fast.

 By the summertime, there wasn't much I could do without having to sit down. I was miserable. I got good at masking the way I felt until my lips and eyelids were dark, and my legs were too heavy to lift no matter what I did. But even with going on, I still found a way to make the best of my life. I was only 34, right. Everything about me changed. I refused to wear my heart disease on my sleeves as though it were a crutch holding me back. In 2013, I wrote Bruised but Not Broken and published part one. I found peace in writing about what I'd seen growing up (through my older sister's eyes). It's raw, but it's the truth. My sales did so well I made that series a trilogy. Instead of going out and being reckless, I learned to stay inside and bury myself in my new hobby.

The regimen Dr. Petracek had me following lasted long enough for my heart overall worked for almost seven years. But in fall 2014, my body couldn't take it anymore. Everything started declining. I was blessed because Dr. Petracek was paying closer attention than I thought he had been.

At my spring follow-up appointment, he asked one of his nurses to work me down the hallway as far as I could go. I made it almost 20 feet before I started feeling light-headed, chest tightened, and I was gasping for air. At that visit, he knew I couldn't make it much further. He explained that it was time to have both valves replaced, but he needed to meet with Cardiac surgical teams to establish a more decisive plan. There is one incident that sticks out in my mind clearer than most. Each year like clockwork, DeWayne and I spend the Christmas holiday with my in-laws. We were all in the family room singing and fooling around like usual. One minute I was teasing the kids about a song on the radio. We danced for one minute. I was dancing, and literally seconds later, I was bent over, grabbing my chest, feeling as though I were about to pass out. My movements must have gotten everyone's attention. They stopped talking and laughing and rushed to where I was standing with the kids.

THIRD SURGERY

In 2015, I felt like my life was about to end. It seemed like no matter what I did, and it wasn't enough. No matter what my doctors wanted me to do, I did it. I changed my medications, regimen, and lifestyle, but my heart was getting weaker.

I couldn't understand why I was back to square A. I'd undergone surgery after surgery, but nothing worked.

Why was I being punished?

It felt like God was. I found myself depressed with no desire to go out and do anything or see anyone. I didn't care about being around healthier people than me, living life with no restrictions or a care in the world. I found myself delving further into a depression without an end in sight. I was emotionally disconnected, spiritually torn, physically tired, and mentally drained. Everybody was telling me to go to God and seek refuge in him. It was hard. Each day after work, I would sit for an hour or two with my bible in hand, reading and writing verse after verse, but nothing helped. I was lost.

I found myself constantly wondering if God loved me or why does he hate me so much? Was there a God at all?

  As time went on, I was sure I had the flu, pneumonia, or an upper respiratory infection, and taking an antibiotic just in case I had an infection. It felt like I was back at square one. The rattling of my chest came with always trying to clear my throat, but nothing came up.
From there, things started getting worse. The fluid I was trying to cough up was blood that was overloading my lungs. I'm not sure why, but neither of my doctors explained how or where the fluid goes.
It took me researching on my own when the valves of your heart leak, the extra fluids have to go somewhere. In most cases, 9 out of 10 times, instead of the fluid being excreted, it settles in other orifices of the body. In my case, the extra fluid settled in my lungs, stomach, and legs.

I was at work at about ten in the morning. I felt light-headed, but I'd gotten used to feeling fatigued, so I didn't think anything of it. I stepped out of the pharmacy to go to the restroom. When I walked back into the pharmacy to sit down, I fell out at my workstation while trying to sit down. I scared my boss and the patients at the cash register. I had no idea what happened until I heard my supervisor Dontell calling my name, but I couldn't move. When I came to, he told me I'd lost consciousness for about a minute or two. I was cognitive enough to call my husband so he could meet me at Methodist Germantown Hospital.

The ride from South Memphis to Germantown was excruciating. My body was fighting against me. Getting an IV was the worse. My body was cramping and spasming at the same time. By the time I arrived at the hospital, I was sure I was dying. After being triaged and having my blood drawn, I couldn't straighten my legs or my arms. It took a little over an hour for my labs to come back. The most electrolytes for me were my potassium and magnesium, which were all critically low. The attendant for that evening explained everything and had me admitted. I did not know your potassium could cause dizziness, breathing difficulties, headaches, palpitations, clamminess, spasming, cramping, and a lot more which triggers my WPW. In a nutshell, all of that coupled with the WPW overworked my heart, causing me to faint. It felt like I was in the hospital for a month, even though it was only four days. After being discharged, they advised me to make a follow-up appointment with my primary cardiologist, which I planned to do. The following morning, I called Dr. Basco's office, hoping to get a same-day appointment.

I was scheduled at 2:45 that afternoon. I didn't have to wait at all. I took a deep breath when I heard Dr. Basco at my exam room door.

Dr. Basco came into the exam as he always does.

"Hi, Charnique, tell me what's going on."

After going over everything with him, he said, "Charnique, I think it's time for you to make an appointment with Dr. Gooch's office.

My heart sank. I said, "what, why?
What's going on, Dr. Basco?
As he looked up, the expression made my heart skipped a beat.
Dr. Basco said it looks like the left side of your heart is getting worse, and there is a significant amount of valve leakage from both your mitral and tricuspid valve. If I were honest, Charnique, I'd say the leakage is way more than severe now. After looking over all of the tests we did while in the hospital and our difficulties for three months. There is a significant change in your mitral valve and tricuspid valve.
It felt like someone had let the air of me of a sudden. I wasn't surprised. I was scared but happy I followed my first mind and my gut.
I said, Dr. Basco, what does it mean for me?
 I cried and cried as he kept talking.

Dr. Basco, I'm so tired of going through this.

He said, "Charnique, be happy that you came in, and we were able to catch it."

Do you need my office to coordinate with Dr. Gooch's office to get you in as soon as possible?

When I hung up the phone, I tried to hide my emotions. But I couldn't. My supervisor Dontell looked up from reading his newspaper and caught my attention. He told me to step out of the pharmacy and into one of the exam rooms to get myself together. I chose the room I'd been using for my breathing treatments. I laid on the exam table and silently cried. I heard a knot on the door. When I answered, it was my supervisor Dontell, trying to check on me. I was embarrassed. My makeup had to be messed up.

My appointment with Dr. Gooch's office was different from the ones I'd before. This particular time when he walked into the room, his energy was off, and from his frown lines, I could tell he wasn't looking forward to seeing me back in his office for the third time needing another heart surgery. Instead of sitting at the exam table, he asked me to sit beside him.

I sighed.

Dr. Gooch said he received your scans, echo, and other results a few days and after looking over everything, he didn't feel comfortable opening me up for the third time.

I didn't understand him.

Why, Dr. Gooch?

I was confused. Without taking a deep breath, I asked question after question after question.

If you don't feel comfortable opening me up again, what does that means exactly?

Am I supposed to wait and do nothing or roll over and die?

He explained, Charnique, your last surgery was long, and you lost a lot of blood. He said, I don't think I can perform a successful surgery, but I can refer you to a fantastic heart surgeon that mentored me after college.

My heart was about to beat out of my chest. I didn't know what to think.

Dewayne had sat back the entire time without saying a word until Dr. Gooch said that.
DeWayne said, okay, so what do we have to do.
Dr. Gooch went to say.
The surgeon is Dr. Michael Petracek he works at Vanderbilt Heart and Vascular in Nashville. It's three hours away but worth the drive.
Crushed was an understatement. I didn't know what to think or what to do. Luckily, I was able to get an appointment for two weeks out.

When I first met Dr. Petracek, I thought he was just another quack doctor. He was an older white man in his late 60's that was borderline deaf in one ear. But after my appointment, my opinion of him changed 100%. He was on point with the technology to make him. Vanderbilt has equipment other hospitals dreamed about. He told me to give him and his team until the following Friday to develop a plan.
What could I say?
Dr.Petracek listened to my fears, hopes, and my dreams during my visit. He told me surgery might not make me feel better, and my symptoms may not change after surgery. I still wanted to believe there was hope for me. If it hadn't been for my

husband, I would have forced Dr. Petracek's hand and had surgery the following week. The period between me becoming Dr.Petracek's patient and my having open-heart surgery was seven years. That was a lot of time. Part of his plan was to increase my exercise program to drop another 15 pounds because he felt it would take a lot of pressure off my heart. His analogy was to imagine placing an engine from a pinto truck inside an eighteen-wheeler and expected it to perform. He'd say it'll work for a short period, but eventually, it will give out and die. The same thing goes for my heart goes for in my adult life. I'd gone from weighing approximately 145 pounds now I'm 185 plus.

Dr. Petracek changed all of the medication doses and added some as well. He increased Metoprolol 50mg twice daily to Metoprolol 100mg twice daily, Furosemide 40mg twice daily to 160mg twice daily, Spironolactone 25mg to 75 mg twice daily, Chlorothiazide 500mg twice daily and an Aspirin 325mg once daily, and of course, I was still taking Lortab 7.5 three times daily. The majority of the medicines were diuretics, and for a while, I practically lived in the bathroom. Eventually, my body became accustomed to taking that high doses, but my body started excreting all the fluid along with potassium and magnesium while taking high diuretics.

I was lying in bed for a few weeks with no energy or appetite after I started taking the medication. I started having the worst body cramps, and the more I tried to move, my hands and legs were spasming. It scared the mess out of DeWayne. He ran out to the store to get Gatorade and something for us to eat. By the time he got home, I was balled into fetal position crying. No matter what I tried, I couldn't get anything down. After Dewayne called an ambulance as I tried to put on the first thing I could find. The attending nurse stepped back into the room about two hours after drawing labs. My potassium and magnesium were critically low. I was happy they were able to find what was going on but disappointing at

the same time. I hated being in the hospital more than anything else, but if it meant I'd stop feeling like my body was being twisted into a pretzel, I was game.
Ughhhh.

I'd had my follow-up appointment with Dr. Petracek so we could discuss a tentative surgery date or treatment plan depending on the Cardiac Surgery team. My husband and I got bright and early before the sun came up at 3:15 am to get o the road for my 8:30 that morning. It felt like it took me forever to get dressed. I had a hard time catching my breath without feeling like I was about to pass out. We finally made it with only ten minutes to spare. We sat in the waiting area for almost an hour for the nursing staff to call my name to have my weight, blood pressure, and medication lists checked. By 10:30, Dr. Petracek walked in. After making small talk, he got straight to the point. I needed to do a few more tests, but this time, Vanderbilt required because they have better technology, giving a better picture.

He said, "Charnique, your tricuspid valve, and mitral valves appear to be leaking severely, but the Cardiac Team wanted a few more tests.

I was frustrated as hell.

Dr. Petracek called one of his nurses into the room to check my breathing. He had her place the pulse oximetry reader on my finger and led me down the hall. Were made it halfway, the reading was at 55%. Before leaving the afternoon, his Nurse scheduled another heart catheterization, stress test, and a TEE for the following Wednesday and a class I needed to attend. He was hoping to have all my tests read no later than next Friday.

We let him know DeWayne, and I would be sailing out to Mexico that weekend for five days, so if he needed me, he could leave me a voicemail, and I'd call him back as soon as we were back on USA soil.

My husband held me together almost the entire ride back home, trying to be positive.

I knew there was someone out there dealing with a lot more than I was without a resolution. I needed to be happy and grateful to have another chance. Even though I'd had two previous heart surgeries, Vanderbilt required all of their surgical patients to attend the introductory class that would only take an hour at the most. I was surprised to see only myself and another young man with his Mom. The young man's name was Jacob. He introduced himself after hearing me talking to Dewayne. Jacob was 23 years. He'd had two previous heart surgeries as well and a pacemaker. I was shocked because I would have expected something like that to be older than he and I.

I knew then if Jacob could go through it, I could. We'd both undergoing open-heart surgery at the same time, just in two different operating rooms. Jacob had his mitral valve replaced with a prosthetic valve. I already

I cried and cried until it felt like my body had nothing left. We drove to and from Nashville for a total of six hours and in the doctor's office for three hours. My body was hurting from the car ride, and my nerves and emotions were everywhere. It took Lortab for pain and a Xanax for my nerves to me down.

The following Wednesday, I had back-to-back appointments. We checked in at 6:45 that morning to the cath lab. My Nurse that morning was Ms. Felicia, and she was God-sent. They had her boggled down with six patients. It amazed me how poise, patient, and attentive all of us were. I knew I was a handful with a limited number of veins that run all over the place whenever they needed to do an IV or draw blood. I was surprised when she only needed one try to do both. I was able to complete all of the tests except for the stress test on the treadmill. I was barely able to walk ten steps without having shortness of breath. Even though it was hard as hell for me to fight through shortness of breath, chest pain, lightheadedness, and fatigue, I pushed through and made the best out of our vacation. In the back of my mind, I kept thinking, "if it was meant for me to die, I wanted to have fun with my husband while I could. We had a blast touring the Mayans in Catalina, Canun, Merida, Mexico. It was so beautiful, and there was so much history that I never knew existed. Dr. Petracek called and left a message just as he promised, even though I couldn't access it until we made it back to land.

As soon we docked in Los Angeles, I turned my phone on to retrieve Dr. Petracek's message. He left his cell phone number to call him. Due to the HIPPA law, I knew he wouldn't be able to say much on the voicemail, so I decided not to check my voicemail until we made it back to our hotel to reach out. The message was straightforward. He said, "Charnique, as expected, things are worse than before. Give me a call back when you're free.

We played phone tag for two days before we were to speak. Dr. Petracek explained, "your Mitral Valve and Tricuspid Valve both needed to be replaced as soon as possible." The leakage is worse than it showed in the previous scan taking by Dr. Basco's office. I was hoping you could call my office first thing Monday morning and ask to speak to Ms. Carol in Cardiac scheduling.

Monday morning came sooner than I would've liked it to. After speaking with Carol, we agreed on June 14, 2015, at 6:30 that morning, with check-in at 4:15. Although I tried my best to hold myself together because I was at work, that didn't work out. About ten minutes after I hung up the phone with Carol, I was in a patient's room with the door closed, crying my heart out. I couldn't understand why it was happening to me at 35. I was about to have my third open-heart surgery.

Why was God putting so much on my shoulders?

Hell, to be honest, I questioned there being a God.

I knew I'd have to have another surgery, eventually, but damn.

The one thing in the world that I consistently asked "GOD" for he denied me time and time again. My faith was wavering more and more.

After agreeing on a date with Carol, I called my husband to talk me through and calm me down.

Was God giving up on me?

I felt like my world was coming to a complete halt. Everything was moving was going fast but slow at the same time. After choosing June 15, 2015, I immediately took off work two weeks before my surgery for my surgery date. I knew from experience I had to try and get my mind together to pull through. Despite everything that was going on, I still found a way to hide my depression. I was so tired, and over everybody telling me to keep my head and to pray.

Only one person knew what I was going through day in and day out, and that person was my close friend Caysen. At least, I think I was able to hide a lot of it from DeWayne. I was tired of praying, being positive, and wearing a brave face for everybody else when I wanted nothing more than to fall apart. The weekend before my surgery, Dewayne tried everything to make sure I felt loved and stress-free.

My Mom and her husband came into town that Saturday afternoon to help me get my house and everything in order. One of the things I loved about Vanderbilt was during the class I attended. They showed us pictures of what we'd go through during surgery and what to expect when we woke. Unfortunately, the hospitals in Memphis didn't offer anything like that. The hospital I had my two previous surgeries, Baptist East Memorial, gave me a brief overview of my first open heart surgery and nothing for the second.

Monday morning, everyone was up and ready at 3:00. I was definitely on edge. Even though I knew what time we needed to leave home for some reason, I still took my time sanitizing and doing everything Vanderbilt required me to do. When we arrived, I had to rush and check-in and finish the paperwork needed by the billing department. I don't think I'll ever understand why patients had to arrive 3 hours before the scheduled time for surgery. It gives me too much time to think about what could go wrong. As I was checking in, my Aunt Carol and my younger cousin showed up. I was surprised and happy to have more support. I couldn't stop the tears from falling down my face. It took almost two hours for them to call my name for transport. My family stood and gave their well-wishes as DeWayne, my Mom, and I was led to the back for pre-op by one of the Nurses from cardiac surgery.

As I expected, the nursing staff was so polite and understanding of everything I needed. It was funny as always. The nurses are so used to older men coming in without shaving everywhere except their heads and showering they were happy to see I followed instructions. After giving me the once over, they allowed Dr. Petracek and his surgical staff to come in and introduce themselves. Dr. Petracek came in first. I should have known then that he was a joker.

That was his first time touching my breasts without a bra. He bucked his eyes and stepped over to the side of my bed.

He said, "are those your real breasts"?

It threw me off for a minute, just as he asked one of his colleagues to come over and see my breasts.

I brushed it off, made light of the situation, and answered his question as I chuckled. Yes, they're mine.

My husband could sense me getting irritating and changed the subject by introducing himself to the other doctor. After they left the room, Nurse Towana told me that I had a few minutes before the anesthesiologist team returned to give me some medicine for my nerves. I had fifteen before they'd roll be to my surgical suite. When my husband turned the corner to get my Mom once last, I let the tears I'd been holding back fall down my cheeks.

I was tired as hell and terrified about going through another heart surgery.

Like clockwork, my surgical team came down to my room precisely fifteen minutes later, smiling at my husband and me. As they rolled me down the hallway, I squeezed DeWayne's hand harder than I had ever before. He kept repeating over and over, Baby, I'll be right here waiting for you to wake up. As soon as they rolled into the room Dr. Janson, the anesthesiologist, asked, "how are you feeling, Charnique"?

I can't lie. I'm scared I need something else to calm my nerves. The only thing that kept running my head was I almost died during my last heart surgery, and I didn't want that to be the outcome.

She did her best to reassure me that I was in the best hands in the United States.

She lifted my IV and gave another 3mls of Ativan as I waited for Dr. Petracek to enter the room. They shifted me, got me comfortable on the table, and turned on some music. I overheard Dr. Petracek say my name right before Dr. Janson told me to take a few deep breaths and count backward.

I woke up in the recovering area before being transferred to my room, scared, feeling like I was in a nightmare. In my dream, someone was chasing me. I'd never seen the man before in my life. He pinned me down and started choking me.

However, my dream felt real to me.

Why or how?

It just did. I dream I'd gotten into a fistfight with the nursing staff who tried to remove the intubation tube from my throat. I started apologizing over and over again, and the Nurses began laughing. I wanted to stop whoever it was from pulling the intubation tube out, but I never tried to fight anyone.

I expected to feel better afterward as I had before, but I didn't. My heart rate started plummeting the following day. At first, the surgical team contributed it me having had heart surgery, but after a few days of my vital bottoming out and racing, they couldn't figure it out.

 I started feeling weaker than I had before surgery. I was scared out of my mind. My Mom and DeWayne were sure it was because I had my diaphragm repaired during surgery and in surgery for almost 16 hours.

Late Wednesday afternoon, the nursing team removed the tubes from my neck and the breathing tubes from my abdomen. Why do things that seemed to be so simple, so hard?

After sitting me up in bed, they instructed me to take a few deep breaths. Then, I felt a tug and a pull on my third exhale, followed by a popping sound. I've had breathing tubes before, but this time before. It hurt like hell. My throat was on fire.

I asked what was different.
After a brief explanation, I had a better understanding. The pain in my throat was from the scar tissue from this surgery and previous surgeries, the new incisions, and the diaphragm.
My stats weren't getting any better.
All of it hurts like, if anyone says it doesn't hurt, they are lying plain and simple.
 My Nurse came in later that night to see if I wanted her to remove my catheter. Once that came out, I felt a little relief immediately until I couldn't urinate on my own. My bladder felt full.
She explained that it was expected, in most cases, but it takes a minute in a small number of patients.

Having heart surgery at Vanderbilt Hospital was different from Baptist East Hospital in Memphis. Cardiac patients are assigned a cardiologist team that follows patients during and after surgery and throughout their inpatient stay. Since my surgery was

on Monday, I expected to be discharged and on the road no later than Saturday.
  Unfortunately, I felt light-headed after Wednesday night, and my heart rate didn't go higher than 50bpm. I could barely keep my eyes open. I was scared out of my mind. One minute my heart rate would rise in the sixties. The next minute, it was plummeting down in the '50s and lower. The ECG monitor that keeps up with the vitals for each patient started going off constantly. I didn't know what to do but to listen to my Nurse's advice. For some reason, the only thing that made sense to me was controlling my pain and the medication they gave me. I knew a little bit from Anatomy and Physiology in college, and if my body were to become too relaxed, my vitals would drop even lower. I had everybody that was there with me on edge. Things started taking a turn for the worse that Friday afternoon. Dr. Petracek visited me every day once I was more coherent to reassure me that my surgery was a success and that my heart just needed to rest.

So on that Thursday, I was stayed up after the phlebotomist did her runs. I could hear him coming down the hall. When he stopped in front of my room, I sat straight up in the bed and spoke before he could finish saying my name.

On Friday, he was concerned with my chest pain and how often I had it. He said it was normal for most patients to experience dull chest pain as their heart was starting to heal itself. But nothing like what I was feeling.

Late Friday afternoon, one of the cardiologists, Dr. Anthony, came into my room and asked if he could talk to me and, if possible, walk with him around the nurses' station.

I told him, "I'll let you know now I have a problem when it comes to pushing myself. I'll always finish whatever the task is. And right now, it's walking around the nurses' station. I'm going to do it no matter how I feel.

Dr. Anthony said, " can this be one of those times when you don't, and I'm trying to see something.
That doesn't sound good.
Is there something else going on with me?
I made it half of the way around before I had to stop and sit down.
Dr. Anthony's expression changed. After I sat down, he placed one of his hands on my wrist, and the other was on my neck.
 He said, I'll be honest, Charnique.
But before I say anything, I need to try to stay calm.
He paused, I think your heart is failing. You may be going into complete or partial heart failure, but he needed to be sure. I stood up with his help. I couldn't comprehend what he'd just said.
I took a deep and tried to make it back to my room without stopping.
I was three doors away when tears started rolling down my face. Before I sat back down on the walker he'd given me, I noticed someone looking at me. It was Justin. He smiled and nodded his head.

The closer I got to my room, I couldn't hold my tears any longer. My Mom must've felt my presence before she could see me.
She came into the hallway to console me before asking, " do you want me to go and DeWayne"?
All I could do was shake my head "yes."
I crumbled when he walked into the hallway.
Dr. Anthony explained what was going on to DeWayne. I sat there feeling like the walls were closing in on me.
I could hear Dr. Basco's voice a few years back. He said, Charnique if you don't have surgery soon to correct your valve problems, you will not live to see 35. That stuck in the back of my mind for years after he said it. One week after work, I stopped by my Grandmother's house, hoping to settle my emotion while checking on my Dad. My Grandmother had always been so good at reading a person's spirit, and that day was no different than any other time. After listening to me go on and on about everything that was happening with me.

The first thing she said was, " now, baby girl, you have that Mack blood is going through your veins. That Mack blood makes you stronger than most people. You need to stand up with your back straightened and hold your head up high. Any and everything that comes your way will only make you stronger.
I played that over and over in my head as I tried to calm myself.
Why me?
Dr. Anthony then looked at me and grabbed my shoulders. I felt like I was about to pass out.
He asked me to explain exactly how I was feeling.
So I did the best I could.
I told him I felt the same as the past few months. I felt faint, lightheaded, and I had chest pain. The chest pain felt kind of like someone was twisting the muscles in my chest into a knot.

When I looked into his eyes, I knew he wanted to see why it was happening to me

just as much as I did. I felt as though I'd
been waiting forever, even though it was
only an hour by before Dr. Anthony stopped
by my room again.
He explained that he couldn't guarantee an
on-call electrophysiologist willing to
perform surgery because it was so late on
Friday.
I wanted to scream at the top of my lungs.
Why couldn't anything be easy for me?
What was I supposed to think? I was 35
years, and my heart was failing.
Once I was back in bed, I couldn't help but
laugh out loud.
I said, Baby ", how could Dr. Basco have
known?"
Dewayne looked just as clueless as I was.
 He said, " I'm lost.
 What are you talking about?"
You don't remember?
Years ago, when I first found out I had heart
problems, Dr. Basco said, "Charnique, if you
don't have your valves replaced, you will
not see 35. I didn't understand or believe

him. There I was three weeks before my 35th birthday, about to die.

How could he have been so sure?

My heart felt so heavy, and there was nothing I could do about it but wait. I felt helpless, scared, tired, weak, and in pain at the same time. But there was nothing I could do except wait to hear from someone.

After getting settled back in my room, my Nurse attached the Telemetry pads to my chest and abdomen, and the machine started beeping. My heart rate was in range for no more than 10 minutes before the EKG and ECG machines began beeping again. It kept happening. It was getting on my nerves. I made everybody, including the kids, promise to keep me awake the entire weekend no matter what happened.

I could see the worry lines in everybody's face, but they agreed. My Mom looked just as scared as I was, if not more. I felt bad because we'd been there for almost a whole week, and Dewayne hadn't left my side. The only time he left me was to go to the cafeteria. I had to beg him to go to my Mom's hotel room to shower and take a nap.

Before he left, my Mom had to promise to call him if anything happened, no matter how small. She pulled her chair directly beside my hospital to be sure she didn't miss anything while DeWayne stepped out to take a shower and change his clothes. My Mom and I watched the movie with Dewayne Johnson starred in San Andreas. Before the movie ended, DeWayne was walking into the room.

 I would have never thought I'd have such a caring man by my side through it all. Saturday was the longest day I thought I'd ever had to go through. My family was just as concerned as I was and had no problem trying to make sure I didn't nod off. It was hard as hell. They were more concerned with my pain level. We watched movie after movie to take away from what I was going through. I hated seeing the look on my girl's faces each time my monitor would go off. Everybody's head would snap back to look at the screen to see how low my heart rate had gotten. They were scared, and so was I. My oldest niece/daughter, yep, that's not a typo. My husband and I raised my nieces for one of my older sisters while dealing with what she had to. I won't get into why that's another story.

My pain on a scale of one to ten was a ten, but I loved me, and there was no way I do anything other than what I'd decided to do. I hated feeling helpless and weak. Most people would think I'd be better with asking for help because I'd gone through the same thing twice before. But asking for help doesn't easier for those that are independent like me. When I say my surgical team and nurse's staff helped me make it through, there wasn't much that happened during those few days after having my heart surgery that they missed. Saturday evening, after everyone, left DeWayne and I settled in, hoping for a bit of silence so I could relax. Around nine or ten o'clock, I was sitting in my hospital when I felt a few heart palpitations, chest pain, and lightheadedness. My machine started beating nonstop. I remember trying to talk to DeWayne, but no words would come out. When he stood to come over to where I was, his face looked flushed, and his eyes turned brown instead of green. He rushed into the hallway for help, and within seconds my Nurse came running into the room. I knew something was wrong. I was scared out of my mind.

Was I dying?

The look on DeWayne's face had me on edge a little bit.

Nurse Tayel ran to my bedside.

She kept repeating, Charnique, You will not die on me, you not die on me. Come on, breathe for me. Open your eyes.

I could feel myself drifting away. I was beyond weak.

If it weren't for my husband calling out to me, I might not have made it.

Baby, baby, please don't do this. When I came to, he and Nurse Tayel were looking down at me, silently praying. It seemed like that night lasted forever. I didn't want to take any medicine that could have possibly make me nod off. I didn't care. I laid in that bed that night and prayed harder than I ever did before. I know I'd turned my back on the higher power, but I was searching for my God. I needed a miracle if I were to live through that weekend.

Knowing what I know now, I started hating and doubting doctors because I knew something was wrong. I knew it.

I didn't understand why I had to be the only one of my father's and mother's children who inherited heart disease when I got prepared to have my first heart surgery. My Dad's sister lied to me and said, " nobody on their side of the family had any heart problems."

My Dad told me he had a heart murmur, but just not to the extent of what I have. I was depressed with no idea of how to pull myself out. The only thing I knew was to talk to my PCP and find a medication to help me cope.

After speaking to him, he prescribed Lexapro and Xanax as Dr. Gooch had done in the past.

It was too much to deal with in more ways than one.

Before leaving the room, Nurse Tayel told me, "I will not lose you, Charnique stay strong for me."

DeWayne came to my bedside with worry lines filling his face. God knows I hated seeing me like this or anyone for that matter. After I'd gone through it before, I thought I knew my limitations, but I was wrong.

Dr. Petracek explained everything about my procedures, and he also said it wouldn't hurt like the sternotomy. There are too many nerves on and around the rib cage to count. No one tells you that when you have any surgery, the nerves are ripped apart. Those nerves are now damaged and have to grow back. Having a thoracotomy is a procedure performed on males. It hurt like hell, but I wasn't going to risk falling asleep. Sunday morning, Dr. Petracek came into see me and promised he'd reach out to one of his friends to make sure I'd get an early slot for my pacemaker.

He said, "Charnique, despite the few complications everything turned out to find. He rubbed my shoulder and apologized for not paying close enough attention to the overall damage to my heart.

 So if you are getting a pacemaker implanted will help you need to have the procedure done.

 Before leaving out the room, he said, "I'll be there looking in on your procedure. That gave me a little bit of comfort even though I was scared out of my mind. I'd never met anyone that younger than with a pacemaker if not for the young man I'd met during our mandatory session.

Finally, one of the Nurses from the surgical team came into my room late Sunday morning to tell me I was to the schedule, and my physician would possibly be Dr. Pablo Saveedra. I had the same restrictions, nothing to eat or drink after midnight, and I'd only take my heart medicines tomorrow morning. At 11:30, I asked for some ice cream, chicken quesadilla, and french fries, hoping I'd stay full while I waited for my to come up for surgery. Unfortunately, I knew there was no way I would eat 1/4 of any of it because my throat was still hurting.
I waited and waited for my name to close to be called Monday morning. The lab technician came like clockwork at 4:30 labs and again two that afternoon. I watched the clock like I was on death row. Four o'clock went by right along with 5:00, 6:00 still nothing. The phone finally rang at 9:00. The nursing staff said they'd be rolling into surgery at 9:15. Dr. Saveedra came into the

suite briefly to check my wristband and left out just as fast. It may have taken him ten minutes to come back. Dr. Saveedra walked directly to the table and asked the Nurse for a scalpel.
I was confused as hell. He was about to cut me without me being sedated.
I looked up at him and said, "stop."
The look on his face was worth a million dollars. He couldn't believe he had almost messed up.
I heard him whisper to the Nurse, questioning her as if it were her mistake.
I took a deep and looked back up at my anesthesiologist Dr. Niang. She bent down close enough so I would be the only person to hear her. She said, "Charnique, I got you. Don't worry.
When she stood up, she told me, "she would be pushing Propofol through my IV after she gave me two doses of Midazolam, Diphenhydramine, and another dose of Alprazolam five minutes after I've dozed off.
Just as she said, I counted to ten even though I'd never made it ten.

Two hours later, Dr. Niang and Dr. Saveedra woke up, letting me know my pacemaker implantation was successful. I remember talking a mile a minute while I rode the elevator up the cardiac floor. As she pushed me back into my room, I was already calling my husband's name. I hadn't felt that good in years. I had energy, but more than anything, I was hungry as hell. DeWayne was so happy to see me. His eyes turned green when I was rolled back into the room. He must've heard me in the hallway talking about food.

When I got close enough to him, "he asked what I had a taste for?"

I knew he would've brought me the moon if he could have.

Even though my throat was sore as hell, I didn't care what he brought back or where he'd gotten it.

I tried my best not to because everyone was feeding off my energy.

But tears flooded my face when he left out that door. I was so happy to have another chance to live and share my story, no matter how long it may last. Yet, I felt a small part of me changing when I rolled out that operating room. I was determined to share the trials and tribulations I deal with daily and bring awareness to incest, molestation, and rape.

And surprisingly, I did.

After having the thoracotomy, my right side hurt like hell. Everything

Dr. Petracek told me it was a lie unless you're a man, that is. On my third day, I was lying in bed when Dr. Petracek's nurse Carol and a nurse from the cardiac team came in. After speaking and asking if I was having any issues, I promised having breasts causes it to hurt much worse than he'd said.

Trust me.

He chuckled and promised to see me later that night or first thing the following day. The expression on my face made. Not long after Dr. Petracek left, my nurse came back with my new dose. They upped my pain medications and made sure it was going around the clock. There was one thing I appreciated Vanderbilt doing, which was they sure each cardiac patient went to rehab and walked the unit two to three times daily.

To me, it encourages patients to get up and get moving. My surgical team stopped my rehab because my heart was racing fast as hell one minute, and the next, it was plummeting.

While at physical therapy, I bumped into the young man I'd met in my training class. That gave me hope, just knowing he'd been through the same surgery I'd undergone.

I can't lie. There were so many months before having surgery that I had a lot more bad days than good. Some morning after, I showered and dried off. I was exhausted. I became unable to tie my shoes, comb my hair, or brush my teeth without sitting down. And because of the WPW, things got a lot worse. I had to pay attention to myself. There were times when I'd blackout while driving or constantly blinking my eyes just to stay awake.

Every day, at the end of my shift, I had to call and talk to someone to keep me awake.

Looking back, I know I could have hurt myself and possibly someone else. But my pride got in the way. Unfortunately, being a black woman, I am not good at asking anyone for help.

The following two days went by without any problems. My heart rate stabilized, the fluid on my legs and ankles starting to come off, and my only complaint was being in pain. As they walked out of my room, I asked if I could go home.
Dr. Petracek turned and told me he wanted me to stay at least two more days before discharging me. When Tuesday morning rolled around, Dr. Petracek stopped by at 4:30 that morning. Of course, I was happy as hell to see him. I was so ready to leave that I didn't hear anything except for those four little words, " can I go home."
In retrospect, I remember walking past some of the other hospital rooms, and now I can see how fortunate I was to have a room full of family there with me.

It was finally time for me to be released. I was scared and happy at the same time. When the nurses there for me came into my room to give me well wishes and make sure everything was okay. I still had questions.
I did. I explained that Dr. Petracek asked if I wanted to try one of the newer drugs before having surgery.
 I think I said "no" before he could finish his sentence and explained why.
I told him, " I work in a pharmacy, and I process all of our recalls for a lot of the newer drugs that have flooded the market. I can't risk it. I understand that it means I'd be on blood thinners for the rest of my life and have to either have my fingers pricked or blood drawn. I'm cool with that. The positive is that I'd know how thin or thick my blood is rather than guessing while taking Eliquis or something similar that doesn't require blood work of any type.
The Nurse from the Coumadin Clinic came in with more information to discuss with my husband and me.

She explained my INR levels were to stay without 2.5 to 3.5. Anything below the 2.5 would mean my blood was too thick and above 3.5 would be too thin.

I'd have vitamin K restrictions. I had to follow a strict diet with a bit of wiggle room. As she explained, I felt dumb. I should've known that Vitamin K would usually be found in green leafy veggies but also fruits. The downside was when the season changed to spring, my husband and I planted our garden. We had kale, lettuce, spinach, and cucumbers.

Ugh.

All of which were all the things I wouldn't be eating until I've found a balance. Everybody in the room started laughing. I didn't notice I'd said it out loud. It was a lot to take it. Keeping a diary of my daily intake wasn't going to be an easy task. But if I was mindful and attentive after four to six weeks, I could start putting more vitamin K back into my diet.

After spending hours researching, I found that keeping my PTT/INR level within range had to be consistent. So to make it simple, if I wanted to eat a salad, I had to pick one day out of a week every week, which made sense.

Every morning I'd lay awake in my hospital bed fighting back the tears that seemed to find a way out no matter how hard I tried to hold them in. I laid there thinking over the months prior. Finally, although I was still in disbelief, I made it through.

How could I walk around every day with my heart failing?

Granted, I'd undergone two previous heart surgeries, but nothing could've prepared me for what I'd gone through within seven days. I had two invasive heart surgeries. Why me?

The drive back from Nashville was a breeze. I promise you the last dose of morphine they gave me before they rolled me out of the hospital had me silly and pain-free. I sang every song and rapped with the radio. I was so happy to be able to have fun like that with my nieces.

When we made it home, I couldn't believe how much they'd gone through to make me feel special.

There was food everywhere. Gail had to have started cooking when my husband called to tell her we were on the road. I had everything I wanted at that moment. My husband was standing, beside me holding me up. My girls were behind me just in case I fell, and my Mom was right behind them. I didn't know how I made it through the last week but having them there for me was enough to make me push myself even harder to get to our routine.

I was so happy we chose to get my prescriptions before I was discharged because I needed them. I used a lot more Lidocaine than I should have to numb my throat that day. After eating nothing at all most days, I wanted to eat and enjoy every bite.

As bad as I wanted to, I couldn't make it upstairs to our bedroom, and that made me mad as hell. It pushed me to work myself hard as hell each day. my first three weeks were terrible. I was frustrated and tired sleeping in my mother-in-law's bedroom because I couldn't make it upstairs to mine. I had none of my stuff downstairs. That was I learned to respect open heart surgery before I'd be out the bed and trying to run around the house. I also had to have my INR checked twice a week. One day it was way too thick, and three days later, it'd be too thin.

Why?

Sticking myself twice a day and going to the lab twice a week was a lot. Most days, I was in too much pain to get out of bed. I wasn't even allowed to bathe for ten days in the first two weeks because I couldn't risk stitches along my side getting wet.

I guess the medicines were in my system more than I wanted them to be. One night during the third week, I woke up feeling like I was on my cycle, but I wasn't. I kept feeling blood clots coming out of me. DeWayne rose to see what was wrong with me.

I looked at him and asked, what was happening to me?

He assured me no matter what it was, and he'd be there with me. He helped me out of bed and into the bathroom. There was so much blood. I couldn't tell if it were rectal or vaginal bleeding until I got into the bathtub. When I looked down, I had clots of blood streaming down my legs.

I panicked, even though this wasn't the first time my hemorrhoids had bled. It was my first time taking blood tinners, and I was already on edge worrying about every little thing.

Once I calmed down, I looked again. It was rectal bleeding because it was bright red. From everything I'd read, Dr. Petracek told me anytime I cut myself or my cycle, it would be worse than anytime before.

What in the hell?

How did it start? I hadn't been straining or done anything to irritate it.
What did I do wrong?
DeWayne asked, was it the blood thinners? No matter how I rationalized it, I didn't know for sure.

I was confused, but there was nothing I could do but wait for it to stop. After DeWayne helped me clean myself up, he helped me back to bed. I was tired of dealing with everything that came with heart disease. I mean, it's not something I'd ever choose for myself.
It was a lot to deal with but giving up was not a choice for me. After all, I had a husband and two little girls that needed me right.
That was a long night with so many more to come. For the life of me, I couldn't find a way to minimize the pain. I knew it had only been a few weeks, but I was impatient. I wanted to be healthy right then.

If there was one thing in this that I hated more than anything, it was to be wholly dependent on someone else to care for me. By my fourth week of being home, I was ready to get moving so I could stick to the plan Dr. Petracek placed me on. For me, contacting St. Francis Rehabilitation center n Park Ave was the best decision I could have made. My husband and I changed eating habits ad adopted a workout plan that worked for both of us. The first three weeks were tough as hell. I started out having to walk at a low speed at 1.2 on the treadmill. Each session, there was a heart monitor and electrodes I had to wear. I didn't think it showed anything until I pushed myself too hard, my heart rate was over 130, and I was dizzy. After that episode, Sue made sure to explain what the monitor did and how, in lamen terms, it monitored my heart rate, pulse, oxygenation, and rhythm.

My trainer noticed I had too many arrhythmias back to back.

She called my name, asked how I was feeling, and asked to step off the treadmill for a few minutes.

 After sitting down for a little over two minutes before trying to explain the pulling sensation on my left side during rehab, even though I didn't want to, I had to follow protocol to sit down and drink some cold water. It felt like it was right underneath my pacemaker, if not in the same spot but different from the shocking it did when my heart rate wasn't within range.

After making my appointment with Vanderbilt, I sat in complete silence and took a minute to do what many people call a self-inventory. I needed to know if there was something I was doing wrong. I sat, I cried, and I sat some more. When I got up, I had a plan. I was going to increase my workout plan and stick to the diet restrictions. Early Monday morning, I reached out to one of Dr. Saveedra's nurses, Trina, for an appointment to ensure there wasn't anything wrong.

At my six-week follow-up appointments, I had three back to back. I thought everything was going great until I made it to Dr. Saveedra. When I entered his exam room, I sat in the recliner next to the computer mounted on the desk. As I got comfortable, the nurse grabbed the monitor and placed the probe directly against my skin.

After taking a few deep breaths to steady my heart rate, I felt a few shocks as it started to read. It was cool. So each time my heart rate dropped below 50bpm, the pacemaker was activated, which sent a shocking sensation similar to jump-starting a car as the probe started reading it like someone was pulling and tugging at it in my heart.

I was scared out of my mind wandering about how the appointment was going to go. When Dr. Saveedra came into the room, I smiled as he shook hands with my husband. I didn't breathe until he sat down next to us. The look on smile his face was reassuring enough to calm my anxiety when

I raised concern about the radiating pain and pulling underneath and around my pacemaker.

I went on to explain. Dr. Saavedra, each time I moved my arm and hand, I told him it feels like the muscles in my chest were being ripped apart. It felt like someone was cutting me with a knife.

Is that normal?

He said he understood my concerns, but because, according to the recording transmitted by my pacemaker.

Not meaning to interrupt him, but it felt like he was dismissing what I was trying to say before I finished my sentence. I told Dr. Saavedra that I understand what you are saying, but is there any way to send me to have an ultrasound. I'd done some research. I knew I'd had pain from the implantation, but nothing like what I was experiencing.

Still, he was reluctant to listen to my concerns. He dismissed my husband and me and walked out of the room. That rubbed me the wrong way.

After six months of going through pain, my symptoms changed and impeded everything I wanted to do. At the time, our master bedroom was on the second floor, which made it almost impossible for me to go upstairs without help. I felt like I was back to square one for the fourth time. The only thing I knew to do was to lose more weight and build muscle mass. I started working at home on the days I didn't have therapy. Even with all of the effort I was putting in, things weren't going my way. I started having more episodes of passing, chest pain, heart rate dropping. I started having bouts of not being to talk and move, but I was able to blink. No one could tell me if it was related to the WPW or not. After a few weeks of going through, I lost my voice again. It was completely gone. I promise you God must've had a unique plan for me. I've always wondered if my testimony was worth all of the pain, persistence, and unwavering mindset of not giving up on me.

Was it worth it?

Would anyone care about a black girl with all of the odds up against her?
Unlike others going through a fraction of what I have, I have the determination and refuse to give up on Charnique.
It had to be around June or July when my heart rate started dropping into the low 50's. There is one day in particular that stands in my mind. I was driving home from work to keep up with the same routine I'd followed after work. I'd call my husband first to let him know I was on my way home. My second was either to my Mom or my oldest sister. I was driving home doing about 70 to 75 miles per hour. I could feel myself getting weak. Coming from work, I felt tired but not too tired to drive myself home. I made it past the Jackson road exits. That evening, I barely had the energy to talk to anybody, so I winged it. I felt myself drifting as I came to, I grabbed the steering wheel as tight as possible. As I looked into my rearview mirror, the cars behind and beside me were at least one-half mile behind. If you've ever driven in five o'clock

traffic, it's usually back up and bumper to bumper. There had to be somebody was watching over that day. I was scared out of my mind. Looking back, I'd had a blackout spell like that in the past. I was taking my mother-in-law to work at the University of Tennessee campus downtown. When I crossed over Poplar, my light was red, but I drove through it. I totaled my car and the young man's that was coming through the intersection.

It took a while for someone to take me seriously when it talked about the radiating pain going from underneath my left shoulder pain, radiating down into my fingers. When my entire arm started getting numb, I knew I had to do something. Somebody had to listen to me. The first appointment I made was to Raliegh-Bartlett Medical Group to see my PCP. From my experience, I learned to always start with your primary care physician first, which for me would be Dr. Thomas Ferguson. After all, he was the first doctor to listen to me. Before coming into my exam room, he had

Margie take me for x-rays just in case I had structural damage. I waited almost two hours, start to finish. Dr. Ferguson did see the wires overlapping on the pacemaker. I never cared about taking medicines for anxiety and depression, but mentally, physically, and emotionally I needed help.
 I'd had my heart surgery about six months before the pain became intolerable.
I called Dr. Basco's office the following day, hoping to get an appointment later that week. When I told his nurse Joanna what was going on, she made my appointment for the same day.
Dr. Basco tried to come up with any excuse he could before sending me downstairs for an echocardiogram, ultrasound, and another stress test. At that moment, I knew I couldn't be like other patients and listen to what my doctor was trying to tell me without researching it myself. I had to wait three days for my results to come back. I felt like those were the longest three days ever.

Dr. Basco's nurse called late Monday afternoon, and I needed to come back into the office as soon as possible. I got there around 9:15 that morning with my nerves on edge. Joann noticed me in the waiting room before calling my name. Instead of going to an exam room, she led me to Dr. Basco's office.

OMG...

What in the hell is going on now.

I could hear Dr. Basco coming down the hallway before seeing his face.

When he entered the room, he said, "Charnique, I found the problem." it looked like the line from the pacemaker was threading through the tricuspid valve. But with saying that, I think it would be best for you to contact Vanderbilt again.

What?

Are you sure?

He simply shook his head, yes.

I thanked him and waited for the nurse to come in to give me the necessary paperwork to take with me to Nashville.

I don't know how but I held it together long enough to it to my car. As I sat there, I punched the steering wheel so many times my knuckles were bleeding. When I made it home, I spoke to our girls and headed upstairs for a hot bath before DeWayne made it home from work. I grabbed my radio, Bluetooth speaker, and my Mahalia Jackson cd. I played Jesus promised me a home over there over and over again. What and how was I supposed to feel?
I stayed in the tub for a little over an hour before heading downstairs to cook dinner. I straightened my back, held my head, and dried every tear that threatened to fail down my cheeks. Even though my family understood most of what I was going through, I couldn't allow anyone to see me cry. I was tired of feeling like I was a burden.
After having my mitral valve, tricuspid valve, diaphragm, and pacemaker implant, I couldn't raise my arms above shoulder levels was way too much for me. I could have done like everyone else and sat home

complaining. But that wasn't in me. Having to jump across those hurdles showed me how strong, determined, and resilient I was. I refused to break. I did the one thing I knew I was good at. I turned my negative health woes into positives. I knew I had a testimony. I just needed to find a way to share it and help someone else.

After being told something else going with my heart could have and maybe should have broken me made me stronger and braver than before. I got up the following day, ready to face the next hurdle laid out for me. After calling and scheduling an appointment with Vanderbilt, I was able to breathe. I'd need to wait for a callback from either Dr. Saveedra, Petrack, or Byrd. It had to be around 4:00 that evening when my phone rang. My heart dropped into my stomach when I looked at my caller ID. I was happy Dr. Petracek made previsions to get me to his schedule for that week. It took a minute for me to want to tell anyone other than DeWayne about my possibility of having another heart surgery.

After sitting and talking with Dr. Petracek and Dr. Byrd, they were sure about me having a few tests done I left that day. Dr. Petracek's pink face turned beet red while he looked at the DVD Dr. BAsco sent him. I could tell by the look on his face he was pissed off after performing an almost 16-hour surgery only months before.
Later that week, I got another phone call from Vanderbilt. Dr. Petracek wanted me to have another heart catheterization and TEE done there in Nashville so he could perform them himself or oversee it.

After having another TEE performed, Dr. Petracek said he'd need to meet with the surgical board before giving me a definitive answer.
I was back in limbo, waiting for someone else to tell me my fate. Luckily without having to call, Dr. Petracek called me early Thursday morning. I could hear the hesitance in his voice. He said there's a problem. The pacing wire coming from the pacemaker was threading underneath and

through your tricuspid valve. And it has been torn almost to pieces.

I sat there and listened as he told me what my next steps were going to be.

As he went on, he said I wouldn't be a candidate to my chest cracked again because it would be too risky. But he'd have an answer by the end of the week, so he wanted my husband and me to come back into the office Friday.

Friday couldn't come fast enough. I felt like my lungs were swimming in the fluid. Anytime I tried to clear my throat, I could hear and feel what I thought was mucus come up to the top of my throat, but nothing would come up. Instead of bothering DeWayne, I waited for him to come home that evening. To calm me mentally and emotionally, I needed to look him in his eyes. If my breathing hadn't been labored, I might have run out of the house to him.

I'm not sure why but I was scared to tell him I needed another heart procedure. I tried hard as hell not to cry, but it didn't work.

That Friday morning, we were back at Vanderbilt, waiting for my name to be called. By 9:00, we were in an exam room waiting for Dr. Petracek. When he came into the room, he didn't look stressed or worried the week prior. After taking a few deep breaths, I was ready to hear the plan to save my life.

He jumped right to it. He said, Charnique, I think we've come up with a plan. Rubbing his knees, he leaned forward and asked, are you ready.

It felt like he was reading my mind, I was ready, but I didn't want the disappointment.

 I shook my head "yes."

Just as he was about to speak, there was a knock at the door. When he opened it, another doctor was waiting to come in. My heart dropped into my stomach. I looked at DeWayne, hoping he knew what was going on. Without saying a word, I sat back in my chair as fear was trying to take over. Dr. George Crossley introduced himself as one of the many electrophysiologists. His demeanor seemed pleasant that often worked close with Dr. Petracek.

After shaking hands, Dr. Petracek cleared his throat and began explaining the reason for his presence. He said there was a procedure performed on cardiac patients that doctors don't believe can make it through a surgery that's already high risk. Transesophageal Valvular Aortic Replacement is referred to as TVAR, but in my case, the valve being replaced or repaired is the Tricuspid. I'd be placed under a light sedation as the surgeon placed the catheter into the femoral artery into the heart to place another valve inside the existing valve. The FDA had not approved the procedure, but they have a pretty successful rate of 85%.

My husband was all for it, although I had my reservations. He insisted on trying the procedure before going with another heart surgery. Partially he felt as though with each surgery, he lost a part of me. After hearing this, DeWayne explains why he felt confident with Dr. Petracek's suggestions. It would be less risky, which I understood. My apprehension was that I was right back on the surgical table nine months later because I had a repair last time. My heart was telling no, but worrying about dying overweighed my feelings.

Once we agreed, they wasted no time calling Tori and Carol, the surgery schedular and Nurse. Dr. Petracek wanted to get my surgery done before he went to have surgery himself. Before leaving that afternoon, we settled on having surgery on August 6, 2017, at 8:30.

I couldn't believe I was going to be back on yet another surgical table to be cut, even if it was a less risky option. There was so much running through my mind. I'd have to get everything I line for my job, with my Mom and the girls. I knew my husband would take care of everything, but the last thing I needed was for him to resent me. I was starting to lose count of all the surgeries and procedures I'd undergone. After having my third surgery in 2015 would have been my last, but no, I was again back where I started. Every bit of faith I had was completely gone.

I knew there was one place I needed to go, that was to see my Dad. I needed the peace that he and only he could provide. A few years prior, my Dad suffered a massive heart and stroke back to back, leaving him unable to speak or talk. While he was in the ICU, the nursing staff kept his hands and legs restrained, which led to the amputation due to their negligence. I'd watched my father lay in bed for years holding on to his life the best way he could. Having to watch my Dad hold on made me fight harder each day.

I went from believing and being thankful for every obstacle I'd overcome to not wanting to hear anyone saying or referencing God. Would God have brought me through three high-risk surgeries just to let me die?

I did what I'd always done. After choosing the date for surgery, the first thing I had to do was coordinate with my supervisor and human resources for approval. It was too much for me to process mentally I was drained. I'd always taken work two weeks before my surgery to gather my thoughts. After sitting at home for a week, I got a call from Tori, Dr. Crossley's surgical nurse. She apologized for calling me early before telling me she needed to push my surgery date back at least three weeks.

Again my heart dropped into the pit of my stomach. I was speechless.

She said Dr. Crossley had broken his ankle and would be out of work for at least three to four weeks for him to get clearance.

I'm guessing Tori could hear the disappointment in my voice. Dr. Crossley told her that he was sure he'd only be out for two weeks even if he had to sit in a chair alongside Dr. Petracek.

Just knowing I'd have Dr. Petracek overseeing the rewiring of my pacemaker and performing the TVAR gave me a moment of peace, even if it was temporary. We talked for at least 15 minutes going through the available dates. It felt like it took forever, but I was finally on the schedule for the third week of August.

I took the extra time off of work to get my life and my mind in order. It was something about having the procedure done that didn't feel right.
I had too much time on my hands to sit and think.
 Like most kids growing up, I remember going to doctor appointments with my Mom regularly. I understand my Mom wasn't a millionaire taking us to our private PCP's but damn.
Why did they do it to me?
Were the doctors that negligent in having never mentioned me having a heart murmur?
The night before surgery, I felt hopeless, helpless, lost, apprehensive, and abandoned at the same time. I'd given my all to stay alive, but the odds were stacked too high against me. As much as I wanted to protest getting out the bed to shower again, wipe down with the antimicrobial wipes, place the Bactroban ointment in my

nose and shave anywhere, there was hair except for my head and eyebrows.

When it was time for us to leave and head to Nashville, I'd done everything I could to put my mind at ease. I was happy as hell when my Mom's husband decided to drive. The entire ride, I laid my head on DeWayne's shoulder, closed my eyes, and pretended to be asleep.

When we were about ten minutes away, DeWayne woke me up. My heart was beating so fast and hard it felt like it had jumped out of my chest. No matter how I felt, I had to face reality after taking several deep breaths as I gathered myself and made my way towards the surgery check-in. As we walked through the door, I heard someone from check-in calling my name, murdering my name, I should say. Catching me off guard, I didn't know what to do other than follow right behind her to her desk. After sitting down, she explained Dr. Petracek and Crossley were waiting for me in the cath lab. Fifteen minutes after walking in, I being led upstairs and piled into another waiting area. By 7:00, I was in preop waiting for Dr. Petracek to come back on the floor.

After switching beds and getting comfortable, I remember lying there questioning my decisions.

Did I make the right decision by listening to Dr. Petracek and my husband?

Will it work?

And if so, how long?

I closed my eyes to gather myself when I heard Dr. Petracek entering the room. When he entered, he said my name and tried his best to calm my nerves. After patting my shoulders, the nurse pushed the Ativan and Propofol.

When I woke up in recovery, DeWayne's face was the first face I saw looking back at me. After making sure I was okay, he left out to get the rest of the family. Before leaving Memphis, my Mom told me my Aunt Carol couldn't make it this particular time. Not only did she come, but she had my younger cousin, Aunt Jam, and her best friend. I wasn't expecting a room full of people looking down at me. My heart smiled.

Shortly after trying to make small talk with everybody, I couldn't breathe. Dr. Crossley rushed into the room as my Mom was running to get DeWayne. All I could hear was my Mom yelling. Somebody get DeWayne to hurry up. Within seconds he was by my side, telling me to steady my breathing. Once Dr. Crossley noticed he knew what he was doing, he rushed out for a breathing machine.

Before leaving the room for the second time, Dr. Crossley sat down next to me for about five to six minutes before saying anything. Without him opening his mouth, I knew what his first question was going after asking me how I was feeling.

I knew he wanted to learn more about what he called bronchospasms. When I was in pre-op, the CNA Latisha working on my units that morning asked if I felt okay or needed anything before my procedure started. I did mention I may need a breathing treatment.

Dr. Crossley asked how long I'd been having problems and how bad.

I hadn't given it much thought other than it started about six months before having my third heart surgery. A few months before having surgery, I could be having a whole conversation with someone, and out of nowhere, I'd lose my breath. Most times, I'd have to sit down and rest before continuing. It happened at work while I was working with a patient. It went from me not being able to catch my breath to chest pain. I remember grabbing my chest before falling to the floor. Luckily, my pharmacist that day was Tamika. She reacted as I collapsed.

I stayed in the hospital for four days without finding the underlying problems other than my heart may have been. I told Dr. Crossley, Dr. Petracek had me see a pulmonary specialist there at Vanderbilt but didn't find anything either. The result was me getting a nebulizer, Albuterol inhaler, Ipratropium, and Albuterol solution.

My three days were finally over, and I was tired of the hospital food and more than ready to go home. I hated I had to keep my left arm in a sling for one to two weeks, all depending on how the stitches over my pacemaker healed and not put any unnecessary pressure on my right leg.

Those two weeks flew by. Even though I hadn't done much with my left arm, I was ready to try.

I'm not sure what I thought my recovery would be, but it was not like the three times before. The TVAR procedure was for Dr. Petracek to enter my heart by threading a catheter through my leg into my heart.

Once inside the tricuspid valve, he attempted to crack the existing valve open enough to slide another bioprosthetic valve inside it.

It sounds simple, huh?

No.

I'm not sure of what I expected to happen precisely. Was I supposed to have the same feeling I had when I came out of the surgery in 2015 or what?

The only thing that seemed better was I
didn't have the pulling sensation that
spread across the left side of my chest
whenever I moved my left arm.
That in itself was a blessing but was that it?
About two months into my recovery, I was
lying on the couch when I started having
the worse lower abdominal pain I'd had. I
dealt with it for a week or two hoping it was
just a muscle strain. Unfortunately, because
it hadn't gotten any better, I called an
OBGYN. It didn't take long for me to find a
name that I recognized, Dr. Kira Cooley.
She'd worked at Christ Community, where I
worked for a few years but had recently left
to start her practice. After being placed on a
brief hold, I was happy to get an
appointment the following week. The pain
became worse, and I ended up in the
emergency room. I had an ultrasound and a
pap smear, they found two fibroid tumors
almost the size of a grapefruit.
I wasn't shocked because my Mom and
both of my sisters have had the same or
similar issues ib the past.

A few years prior, I was diagnosed with having fibroid adenomas covering both of my breasts, so fibroid tumors didn't shock me. After leaving the hospital, I scheduled a follow-up appointment with Dr. Colley's office instead of seeing Dr. Cooley. Dr. Esteep was straightforward about needing them removed because they were more than 10cm in size. She referred me to the West Clinic. I needed to have a biopsy to see if the mass were benign or malignant. The only I heard was benign or malignant. Cancer or not?

What in the hell?

I listened, but my mind was all over the place.

Oh my God. I had a smile on my face, but I was mad, discouraged, hurt, and many other emotions all at once. Dr. Estepp patted me o the shoulder and told me she'd be there with me every step of the way. I was scheduled with Dr. Tillmann the following day at 10:00.

I was happy no one was at home that afternoon. I yelled and screamed at the top of my lungs and cried until I couldn't cry anymore.

During my appointment, I sat there motionless and numb to everything that was going on. Dr. Tillmann did two ultrasounds that day. He found the fibroids and a mass resting on my large intestines. If I could have jumped off the examination table and run out of the room screaming, I would have. I was so over it. I was over life.

Why did it always have to be so hard? After wallowing in doubt, I was up the following day ready to get these things out of me, hoping it would stop me from hurting. Dr. Tillmann's office called two days later instructed me to hold my Warfarin for two days so I could have a biopsy on Monday. I had to get clearance from Dr. Petracek, but luckily he didn't give me a hard time after I explained in detail what was going on.

When I arrived at the West Clinic at 6:30 that morning, I had to get my INR to make sure I was in range. I wasn't. My blood was way too thin, which meant I'd have to wait two more days or be admitted into the hospital for them to regulate my blood using Lovenox.

Ughhh.

The last time I used Lovenox was right the week my Dad died. I was at the wake rubbing my Dad's head when my stomach started bleeding through my shirt. That is not a good memory for me.

I hated using it because it reminds me of losing my Father.

I went through numerous appointments before Dr. Tillmann decided my best option would be to remove the tumors. I decided it would be best to kill two birds with one stone. My husband and I had talked for years about having children until I asked Dr. Petracek completely ignored my question each time I asked if he thought I could start planning to get pregnant. His answer was simple if I got pregnant, DeWayne would have to choose my life or our child.

Initially, I thought he was an arrogant ass, but it made sense. My heart wasn't strong enough to pump enough blood for me and a fetus if I got pregnant. So with that, I asked for a complete hysterectomy after talking it over with DeWayne. It was the hardest decision I ever had to make. I'd always seen DeWayne and me with a house full of kids with his eyes and smile with a mixture of our features. But that wasn't in the cards for me.

It took about two weeks for me to get on the schedule for surgery. I was scared as hell, but I faced it head-on.

I told Dr. Tillmann I would prefer to have my surgery before the end of the year because I'd already met my out-of-pocket and deductible with my insurance after having my heart surgery a few months prior.

It took a minute to get approval from Vanderbilt. Still, after a lot of begging, Dr. Petracek finally caved and gave me the authorization I needed when the surgical nurse called late one afternoon asking if I felt up to having surgery by the end of the week on December 8th.

When she asked, I blurted out " hell yea"
without thinking.
Early that morning, DeWayne and I arrived
thirty minutes before I had to check-in.
Surprisingly, it didn't take as long as I
thought it would. By 9:30, we were situated
in the surgical waiting for my name to come
across the board. Dr. Tillmann's surgical
went over and beyond to ensure I was
comfortable and confident in their surgical
abilities.
My surgery was successful, but the stressful
part was waiting three to four weeks for the
biopsy results to come back. I was on my
way home Sunday morning, and I was
happy as hell. If there was one thing I was,
it was the hospital. Let me tell you, just
because the doctor tells you the procedure
will laparoscopically using what they called
the robot. This method allows the doctor to
make small incisions instead of the bikini
cut. Even in doing so, that does not mean
there will be less pain.
In my mind, it made sense to have surgery
while I was already off of work healing from

heart surgery. I knew if I put it off and returned to work, it would be impossible to take off for four weeks, especially dealing with a whole lot of mess. It took a couple of weeks for a surgery spot to open, but I was able to get in December right before Christmas because of a cancellation.
It felt like my cervix, fallopian tubes, and ovaries had been set on fire and scrapped out of me with a razor blade. Either way, they were taken out. Because I'd had the TVAR procedure, my left leg was already swollen and painful. By doing so, I either slept on my left side or my back. There were a lot of days I'd just about standing on my head trying to alleviate the pain.
A few weeks had passed without the bleeding subsided. I felt like I could pass out at any time.
 So I reached out to Dr. Tillmann's office. When I reached out, I spoke with one of the nurse practitioner's Lyann, if I'm not mistaken. She called ahead and requested me a room at Methodist Germantown just

in case something was wrong. I took my time getting ready.

  After I checked in, the nursing staff took all the blood I felt I had in my body. It didn't take long for my bloodwork. When my results came back, my potassium, magnesium, hematocrit, hemoglobin were all critically low. I expected something to be off but not all of it. Of course, with all of that coming back out of whack, they had to contact Dr. Petracek and Dr. Byrd.
They called at 2:30, and by 3:00, Dr. Petracek was on the phone fussing up a storm. He had a certain way he wanted to be, and he expected it to be followed. Once off the phone with him, Lyann came in. Dr. Petracek told her I needed to have a PTT/INR drawn as well. I had to hold the Warfarin changed be Lovenox and a Heparin drip for two days with a repeat of INR morning and night. If I were to develop a blood clot, it would be fatal.
After being in the hospital for six days, my biopsy results were finally ready. As the words benign left the nurse practitioner's

lips, I felt like shouting out loud as tears ran down my cheeks. I couldn't wait for DeWayne to get off of work was so happy to have something going my way. I felt like a weight had been lifted off of my shoulders. I was back to getting my INR checked once weekly instead of twice a week. Things couldn't have gotten any better.

As the months rolled by, I thought everything was finally working out for me. It was January 2020. I felt good, minus the chest pain and shortness of breath with everything I'd been through over the years. I felt like if that were the only two things I'd have to deal with, I'd be okay. I could deal with that, right. No. I'm not sure what I did, but I couldn't shower, comb my hair, brush my feet, and the list goes on. I had to sit down to do everything just about. There were so many days I'd sat and cried.

If there was a mystical person beyond the clouds, how could they keep letting this happen to me?

 I'd been going through for almost 15 years, and no matter what I did, nothing worked. I could've slapped the excuse my french but the shit out of myself for listening to my husband and Dr. Petracek.

Around May or June, I bit the bullet and reached out to Dr. Basco's office for an appointment.

As usual, I scheduled my appointment on a Friday around the end of my shift. By 3:00, I didn't have enough energy to talk, type, or get out of my seat. I stood and walked out of the door, but I only made it to the triage area right outside the pharmacy. It felt like my body was vibrating, and I had a sharp, piercing pain radiating across my chest as I sat down. I'm not sure how, but I raised the seat enough to knock on the pharmacy door.

Luckily, a nurse was coming down the hall as I almost fell out of my chair. When the ambulance arrived, the EMTs, my body had spasms so bad I couldn't lay still enough to start fluids. That was the quickest I've made it to Methodist Germantown Hospital, or it just seemed fast to me. I had too much hooked up to me and IV"s in both arms. After having labs drawn, they found my electrolytes were causing some of my problems, but the bulk of it was because my heart valves were pumping enough blood. I could've rolled over and given up right then. When my nurse came in to tell me I knew, she thought I was incoherent and not understanding what she was saying. She couldn't tell me anything other than that. I'd have to speak with my primary cardiologist. After getting my electrolytes back in range, I was ready to go. DeWayne and I both sat in the car speechless for a minute. I put my shades on and turned my head towards the window. I didn't want him to think I was weak for crying, so I tried to hide it. That didn't matter. He grabbed my shoulders and forced me to turn around. I wanted to cry like Viola Davis with the snot running out of my nose down to my lips. DeWayne opened his arm and got out of the driver's seat. I didn't know what he was doing. He opened my door and held me. He said, " Baby, I got you."

I knew something was wrong, but I couldn't put my finger on it. That night I cried until there was no fluid left in my body. The following morning, I was back on the phone calling Dr. Basco for an appointment. After talking briefly with Joy, I was able to get in the next day.

At my appointment, I tried explaining everything that was going on. When I left Dr. Basco's office, I felt worse than when I went in. I kept telling him precisely what was happening, but he kept writing it off as symptoms from my previous surgeries. I could barely stand as I stood at the counter waiting for Joy to give the paperwork to have my blood drawn. Dr. Basco caught up with me and asked if I thought about talking to a psychologist because I could be dealing with anxiety and depression. I agreed, but I knew it was something. When Joy made it back to me, I was holding onto the countertop to hold me up. She grabbed a wheelchair and pushed me to the lab. I promise while the young lady was drawing my blood, she pulled every bit of energy I had holding together.

My mother-in-law drove me to the doctor that day, even though I tried to protest against it. DeWayne must've seen the look in my eyes when he insisted on me not going by myself. When Joy rolled me downstairs to the car, I could barely get myself out of the chair and into the car without help. When I made it home, I barely made it inside the house. When I made it to my room, I crawled in bed, fully clothed and balled into a ball. It was maybe half an hour later my body started spasming.

It took me being admitted into the emergency room again for him to understand something else was wrong. This time at my follow-up appointment, he got to see how I could barely walk 2 feet without stopping and exhausted I was while sitting still. I had a heart catheterization, stress test, and a TEE done at the West River location two weeks later.

Instead of Dr. Basco calling as he usually would, he had his Lead Nurse Joy call.

She said Dr. Basco didn't want to deliver the bad news. But I needed to make an appointment with Dr. Petracek at Vanderbilt Hospital because there was a significant change in the amount of fluid coming from both mitral and tricuspid valves. I was mad and happy at the same. The same day, I called Vanderbilt to schedule an appointment with Dr. Petracekand Dr. Byrd. Oh my god, I wanted to scream when the receptionist told me that they'd both retired a few months prior. My new cardiologist and cardiac surgeons were both trained and worked closely with Dr. Petracek, the cardiologist was Dr. Goel, and the surgeon was Dr.Absi. The last thing

I needed was having to acclimated with new physicians.

I had to take a second and calm myself so that I wouldn't be rude. After setting an appointment for the following week, I was on pins and needles.

As usual, when we arrived, the staff was pleasant and attentive to any needs of the patients. About an hour passed before I was called for triage. The medical assistant asked me to follow her and never looked back to see if I was following right behind. When she did, I'd only made it 5 feet. Shortly after getting settled into one of the exam rooms, Dr. Goel entered the room. He had a pleasant disposition, but he was almost age. The first thought in my head was he couldn't have enough experience to know anything about what I was going through.

I was hesitant, but what could I do?

During my visit, I tried to be optimistic after all Dr. Petracek had trained him. What was funny was each time he wanted to ask a question, Dr. Petracek had it written in my chart. After going back and forth with him, he asked me to sit at the exam table, which was fine with me.

When he checked was the swelling of my legs and feet, he said, your feet don't seem swollen to me.

I chuckled, " really." Well, not to be funny, but I'm surprised Dr. Petracek didn't tell you I'm nothing like your other patients. What's typical for them isn't typical for me. Most heart patients hold fluid in the ankles when the fluid pools right below my knee, stomach, and in my lungs.

He stepped back for a second to look again and agreed. I could tell he was thinking to himself. Dr. Goel said, let me check something else. Next, he checked the pressures in my neck surrounding my carotid artery. At the end of the appointment, he changed my medications again. I added another diuretic, Metolazone 2.5mg, twice daily, and increased Metoprolol, Spironolactone, and Torsemide.

Saturday morning, I took the first dose of all of my medications, including the new drug Metolazone. When I say I was tired of urinating, and I was exhausted all the way around. I didn't know what to do. Dr. Goel did tell me to keep a diary to track any weight loss. By Sunday morning, I'd lose 13 pounds. I was shocked I had that much fluid.

Monday morning came too fast when my alarm that morning I couldn't do anything but lay there. I laid in bed for as long as I could. I finally dragged myself out the bed and into the shower right at 7:00 that morning. I'm not sure how I managed to make breakfast and a smoothie, but I did. By the time I made it to work, my body felt like it was vibrating. I wasn't sure what was going on. There was one that I've made my motto while going through my journey. I believe if I sit still and lay around the house, I'd be giving up. I remember sitting at my workstation and laying my head on the counter. My head started hurting, and it felt like someone was squeezing the base of my skull. I stood up from my workstation and tried to walk toward the door. When I made it out of the pharmacy, I leaned against the wall. I was only able to make 5 to 10 feet before sitting down. Everybody that passed me stopped and asked if I was okay, simply because I was embarrassed.

Why?

I hated bringing attention to my struggles with heart disease. At that moment, I had no choice. I'm not sure who caught me as I almost fell out of the chair. All I remember was my body spasming, my pacemaker constantly shocking, and the inability to hold my head up. I could hear someone calling my name and asking me to open my as they carried me to one of the exam rooms. I don't know how long I was unconscious, but Dr. Potter stood beside the exam table, rubbing my hands when I opened my eyes.

When the ambulance arrived, the spasms got started getting worse. I couldn't form my words, but I was able to point towards my medical alert bracelets. If there was nothing I needed them to know, I needed to tell them about my WPW and heart valves. Because I'm a severe heart patient, the nursing staff was waiting for me at the door when I arrived. After I was triaged and on my way to a room within two hours, I knew by the way I was feeling there was no way I'd be going home that day. After rerunning my bloodwork, the charge nurse came into my room and told me I'd more than likely stay in the hospital for a minimum of three days if my potassium and magnesium stabilized. I stayed up the night before my third day. I knew the phlebotomist would come into my room around four that morning. I had everything timed. My results should be by six that morning, and if my bloodwork came back within range, I could go home that morning. That didn't happen. That was when COVID started running rampant in the USA.

It took almost a whole week for potassium to level out. I was taking potassium and magnesium by mouth as well as by IV.

When I did get discharged, I didn't have any veins left to give or get blood.

On Monday morning after being discharged, I first called Vanderbilt and Dr. Basco's office for an appointment. Even though I knew Dr. Basco would refer back to Vanderbilt, I wanted to try at least. Later that afternoon, I received a phone call from Joy, Dr. Basco's nurse. I knew what she was going to say before she opened her mouth. Dr. Basco wanted me to reschedule my appointment until after I've seen Dr. Goel again.

Ughhh.

Dr. Goel's schedule was so full that I had to wait for his charge nurse to call back to get on his schedule. When Wendy reached out, I explained what had happened since my last visit. After explaining why I was rushed to the hospital, she could squeeze me in on the Friday of the following week. I let out a sigh of relief. I let her know I hadn't been able to take the Metolazone, so I was swelling pretty bad. That week was pretty bad for me. I felt as though my lungs were floating in fluid. Each time I inhaled, my chest rattled, making it harder to catch my breath. God knows I wasn't sure what could be done at the time because Covid was starting to ramp up even more. At my last appointment, Dr. Goel went over Vanderbilt's new policy to ensure their patients' safety. They'd had canceled all elective procedures until further notice. Luckily, open-heart surgery was not one of the procedures that'd been canceled.

My appointment was at 8:30, so I was up bright and early trying to shower and get ready. After getting out of the shower, I went into my walk-in closet to grab something to put on. It was about 4:00 in the morning, and I was half asleep. I tried to lean down to grab my pants. I blacked out and hit my head against the wall. I'm not sure how long I was on the floor. When I opened my eyes, it felt like I had someone was pounding on my head. Once I was lucid enough, I walked into the living room for DeWayne. The knot on my head tripled its size. He glanced up without really looking at me. I was dizzy as hell. When he looked up at me, he said, " baby, what did you do." Trying not to fall, I said nothing. I was trying to hurry up and get ready so that we could get on the road. DeWayne was not worried about being late for my appointment. The entire ride to Nashville, DeWayne did whatever he could to make sure I didn't fall asleep. Anyone that knows me can tell you as soon as my body relaxes, I'm out like a light. I've been that way since I had my pacemaker implanted.

That was the longest drive ever. My head was hurting, I was nauseated, and I had chest pain that wouldn't stop. We were only 75 miles outside of Nashville when we heard the tire pop. After calling and getting in touch with Dr. Goel's nurse, I turned my attention to my husband and the tire. It took him longer to get the tire out of the trunk than to put it on the car. We were back on the road within twenty minutes. Dr. Goel made provisions to see me that day. Granted, I had to wait longer than I usually would, I was glad I didn't have to reschedule.

We waited for about two hours before being called back to an exam room with an additional hour wait. Dr. Goel finally came into my room. The look in his eyes when he looked at me was different. When he asked me to sit on the exam table, the walk from the chair I was sitting in seemed like a mile away instead of six steps. On my third step, I had to reach my hands out for DeWayne. As I sat down, Dr. Goel asked if my chest pain had gotten any better and if the Metolazone was working for me? DeWayne tried to explain what was going on because it took longer than usual to catch my breath. That was the first time he took me seriously. Again he placed his fingers against my carotid artery to measure the pressure. He stepped back, and for the first time, he said, "you need to see one of our heart surgeons."

Before leaving, Dr. Goel scheduled another TEE and a heart catheterization for the following week. I was irritated as hell because my symptoms may not have been so bad if he had listened to me. At my last visit, Dewayne was satisfied because I was always trying to get cut open instead of trying an alternative first. My thought process was different, though. I spent a lot of time researching my symptoms and diagnosis. It took us 20 minutes to make it from the exam room to the elevator. I was having excruciating chest pain, and I could barely breathe.

I had my test on the following Monday at 9:30, but it took an additional two weeks for me to get my results. Those two weeks were the worse I'd ever gone through. I didn't have the energy to walk, talk, socialize, comb my hair, shower, or put on clothes.

I was ready to give up. It felt like no matter what I'd done and how many changes I made, I was still back at square one. There were many days I struggled to keep my eyes open at work and during the drive home. My days were work, home, cook, bedtime with a whole lot of hating god and blaming my Mom and Dad.

I got a phone call from Dr. Absi's lead surgical nurse Cassandra to schedule an appointment for a surgical consult. I wasn't sure if my heart was dropping into my stomach or heart palpitations. I had to be back at Vanderbilt Thursday morning at 8:30.

I was already apprehensive and scared out of my mind. I didn't know what to expect, even if Dr. Petracek trained him.

Dr. Absi was straightforward, just like Dr. Petracek.

He said, Charnique, the leakage from both the mitral and the tricuspid valves are both severe. Dr. Absi started flipping through the folder with all of my medical information, looked back up at me, and said, you've been through so much. His first thoughts were I'd been through a lot for someone so young, and he'd love to help me any way he could.

I can't lie. The apprehensiveness was indeed a thorn in my side. I wanted Dr. Petracek and no one else.

Ughhh. Before leaving, I stopped by the cardiac surgery nurse Carol to choose a date for surgery. DeWayne sat and pondered over the schedule for about twenty before settling on September 3, 2020, at 6:00 am. I laid my head on DeWayne's shoulder and silently cried and cried. It took me forever to pull myself together. He held onto me from the elevator to our car. Anybody looking at me would've thought I'd lost my best friend by looking at me. Dr. Absi not only gave me his prognosis, but he listened to my concerns.

During our ride home, DeWayne could tell I was too tired to talk, so he talked enough for the both of us. He went on and on about how he'd make sure I never needed anything as he'd done in this past. That wasn't my concern. My mind was running all over the place. I wasn't sure if I would go through having my chest cracked open for the fourth time.

At work the next day, I started getting my ducks in the row. I had to get the FMLA paperwork filled out and turned in. It felt

like it took me forever to fill the paperwork.
I had to keep stopping. Between the
shortness of breath and the chest pain, I
was exhausted by 10:00 that morning.
Luckily, my supervisors were understanding
and willing to accommodating. My last day
of working was August 20, 2020. I had to be
at Vanderbilt on August 27, 2020, so Dr.
Absi could regulate my PTT/INR. I wasn't
looking forward to it, but what other
options did I have. Was it going to be safe
to have surgery while Covid 19 was running
rampant throughout the world?
The hospital administrators turned the
garage into a triage unit. Dr. Absi and the
staff reassured me that everything would
be fine. I'd have to minimize the number of
people that would be with me from arrival
to discharge. Instead of being in the
hospital five to seven days, it was almost
two weeks. I pouted, but I'd do nearly
anything if I could feel better than I did.
No matter what I did the week before I had
surgery, I was exhausted. After going out
with DeWayne to get everything I needed, I

only wanted to sleep. Through each of my heart surgeries, I've stayed adamant about getting my emotions under control before going into surgery. This time was no different. I was scared out of my mind. It took a lot of encouragement and constant affirmations every day.

The first day being in the hospital with no real restrictions was right up my alley. Other than having an IV in my arm, I was fine. By the third day, I was ready to run out of the hospital. Every morning like clockwork

 I was awake at 3 in the morning when the phlebotomist entered my room. I was more anxious and worried if everything would be okay after surgery than her taking blood. By day five, I was ready to run out of the hospital.

The night before the day, I couldn't have anything to eat or drink after midnight, so I made the best of the choices of restaurants surrounding Vanderbilt. We settled on the pizza place. The nurses raved about this place, Slim and Husky. It was reasonably priced, and Uber eats delivered it. I ate more than I should've, but I was fat and happy. I didn't finish eating until 11:45. When I ordered my food, I ensured the nursing staff didn't bring my medications until ten minutes before midnight. My surgery was scheduled to start at 6:30, so I had to be awake no later than 4:30.

I didn't sleep a wink that night. Yes, I was ready to have surgery, but I was hesitant. I know I've probably said it a million times. I sat in bed thinking over each surgery I'd undergone from the first until the last in 2017. I was 40 years old, and I'd experienced more than most people twice my age. I laid there and cried. For my surgery to be successful, I'd need to calm my nerves and settle my mind.

DeWayne had his alarm set for 5:00, and my Mom and her husband were 20 miles away. I took a few deep breaths and put on my game face.

My Mom came made it right after I'd was transported to the inpatient surgery suite. IWhen she turned the corner and entered the room, I could immediately feel her energy and love. She leaned and kissed my jaw, and it took everything in me not to break down. Twenty minutes later, the surgical team came in the room with paperwork to sign off and introduce themselves. Everyone was friendly, and I loved the energy of the anesthesiologist Tara. She promised to make me comfortable and stay with me from the beginning, end, and three days after because of the severity of my surgery.

If you think I'm babbling, please forgive me. It's been the most challenging book I've written. You'd think, after everything I'd been through, this would be easy, it's not. It's been an emotional battle, and a lot of tears shed putting my thoughts on paper. After being rolled back into a surgical suite, I closed my eyes and asked my God for forgiveness for any and every sin that I'd made. When Dr. Absi came into the room, I called his name. Even though I knew to have a decent scar going down my chest Dr, Absi would have to remove the old scar

tissue. I made sure he knew the plan.
Everybody in the room burst out laughing. I could hear the surgical technician Jessica above my head.

 She said, you are a trip girl. You'll be in surgery at a minimum of 12 hours, and you are worried about the scar going down your chest.

Uh, yeah. I'm still young, and I love to have a little bit of breast showing.

Now that cleared the air. Everybody was laughing. The last thing I remember was trying not to fall asleep as I counted to 10. I lasted until I made it to 7.

I woke up in a recovery suite with DeWayne at my side. My throat was killing me. I looked at DeWayne and shook his head. I asked, "did I do it again, huh."

Laughing, he said, you think.

After having my third open-heart surgery, I dreamed that someone was trying to cut my throat. I have no idea why but that haunted me each time. Each time medical staff would try pulling the intubation tube out of my throat, I'd pushed back in the opposite direction. And the next, I'd be cursing myself out. The pain from not being able to eat or swallowing was the worse. Laying in the hospital bed, I felt better than I'd felt in 16 years before having my first heart surgery. The wires to my pacemaker were changed again, and both heart valves were mechanical.

I'd gotten used to having a mechanical Mitral valve and listening to the constant clicking, getting used to having two clickings sound like a private band at the alternating time. I lost count of how many nights I laid in bed crying. My husband would raise and say, " you need to learn to embrace it and appreciate. And it was his way of knowing I was still here with him. I understood what he was saying. It's just harder said than done.

Many people only understand what they see when a person has open-heart surgery, not the everyday struggle it takes to get back to some type of normalcy.

Immediately after having surgery, patients are put in ICU, where you stay for three to five days depending upon how well you're recovering. Most of the time, I'd say at least 50 to 60 percent of patients fall into depression because there's no one to support them when a person has to become dependent upon someone else to do everything from the smallest to the largest. I opened my eyes to twelve tubes going in and out from my neck to above navel and two breathing tubes from the abdomen. From experience, I had to have someone to hold me upright when I wanted to stand up, walk, use the bathroom and wipe myself. Luckily, Vanderbilt still offered patients and heart pillows to hold against my chest when I tolled over in bed or changed positions, stood, sat down, and coughed. To this day, I still drive with a pillow behind me and one in front of my chest. Allowing someone to have that kind of control over me was the hardest thing for me to do.

After being transferred from ICU to the cardiac step-down floor, I was lying in my hospital bed talking to my Mom. Out of

nowhere, my head started tightening up, and I couldn't move. I could hear my Mom calling my name because I didn't answer her question. She called my name a handful of times, but I couldn't speak. I could hear her footsteps as she hurried to my beside to push the call button. She yelled for help, and a few nurses ran into the room.
The charge name held my name and started calling my name. She needed me to say something and to tell her what was going on. I lost track of how long I laid there, but it couldn't have been more than thirty minutes. Not too long after I settled down, the neurologist came into his evaluation. He asked a few questions before asking if I'd ever had a seizure or anyone in my immediate family had them. I tried explaining my sisters both have episodes, but we all dealt with whatever I had.
The neurologist said he wanted me to wear an EEG monitor so he could capture my symptoms. I think I had the machine on my head for about an hour when I heard Dr.Absi coming around the corner.

When he looked at me, he yelled, "what does she have on her head and why?"
The nurses ran into my room fast as hell. Dr. Absi started ordering them around.
What is that?
Who ordered the device and why?
He made them take the contraption off my head. He fussed for about ten minutes straight. He didn't talk to me until they'd taken it off.
When he did, he fussed at me for allowing them to put it on me. He went on and on about me just getting out of surgery, returning to the nursing station, and fusing some more.
I could hear still hear him ten minutes later. He said before anybody gives me any medication, labs, or other tests, they'd need to get his authorization.
I looked at my Mommy, we both burst out laughing. Everything after that was great. Even the phlebotomist starting changed her schedule to come at a decent. By day four after surgery, it was time for me to start rehabilitation. I wasn't 100%, but I felt good

enough to push myself. The rehab tech tried her best to get me into my room after the first round, so I didn't overwork myself. I told her straight up. Look, I've spent a lot of time lying in bed because it was the only thing I could do. I'm ready to live again. What could she say?

Nothing.

After each exercise, I'd have to sit up in the recliner. I've said once, and I'll repeat it if, for nothing else, I love Vanderbilt because it's mandatory for patients to get up and move.

Day five after having surgery, Dr. Absi and his team came in around 6:30 that morning. He looked over my charts, removed the gauge to check the incisions on my neck, chest, stomach, and inner right thigh. I was happy as hell when he said everything looked great, and he didn't see any reason to keep me any longer. That was music to my ears. I'd been in the hospital for almost two weeks.

To be honest with me, I was scared out of my mind. I'd spent a lot of time trying to find documentation of patients surviving with two mechanical heart valves, not to mention a pacemaker. I checked everywhere but came up empty handy. Dr. Absi made sure I understood how thin my blood needed to be, and there wasn't much wiggle room. I'd have to get my PTT/INR checked twice weekly until I stayed on the thinner side for more than two weeks. The plus side to that was that I'd started using AEL Bartlett after my third heart surgery. Ms. Mattie was always excellent, patient, and kind, no matter how I looked and felt. And she barely had to stick me more than once.

I started having problems swallowing after having my third surgery, as if I couldn't imagine it had gotten much worse the fifth time around.

Having my chest cracked was just as I remembered and much worse.

What in the hell made me do it again?

I was back at square one. I had to depend on my husband, niece, and mother-in-law for everything. My first couple of weeks of being home was anything but a cakewalk. The pain was unbearable, and there wasn't any way to alleviate it other than taking medications.

By week five, I was getting up and out the bed by myself without having much help. I was still unable to bathe myself and comb my hair without help. I'm not sure what I expected, but the amount of pain I was still in was unbelievable.

When I reached out to Dr. Absi charge nurse, she was not happy about me calling for more pain medication. After going back and forth with her for a few minutes. She tried to refer to the laws regarding filling controlled substances for out-of-city patients. I pulled the phone away from my face and laughed.

I asked Carol if you had taken the time to read over my paperwork before returning my call. I've worked in the pharmacy field for over 23

years with many doctor's offices and patients, I'm well versed in pharmacy law. Nowhere in the law books does it say you

can't provide your patients with medications after surgery. And to make her think about what she was saying to me, I told her, " most patients that have never had their chest cracked before that may be true, but no for someone that has had their chest cracked four times prior.
Of course, she wanted to double-check. I didn't have a problem with that or her calling Dr.
Absi. Within a half-hour, she was calling back with her tail between her legs. All I could do was laugh when she called me back.
Dr. Absi called me the following day to check on me and to apologize for Carol's mistake. I brushed it off. I knew she was just doing her job before ending the phone call /Dr. Absi did warn me again about taking the Oxycodone and making sure I wasn't becoming addicted to it. He wanted me to rotate Tramadol and Oxycodone between the two depending on the severity of my pain.

I'd just started rehab, and they were wearing me out. When I first started, Johnathan set a goal for myself from my doctors. At first, I walked maybe 1/4 of a mile at the lowest setting three times a week for two weeks. After my first two weeks, I noticed I was the youngest in my time slot.

I couldn't believe how my hard work was paying off. I was three weeks into my rehabilitation,] I was losing weight and feeling better than I had in years. Don't get me wrong. I pushed myself harder than anyone in my class. I wanted to get back to the old energetic, and painless as possible. Although my rehab sessions were supposed to last 12 weeks, I had to stop at week ten to return to work. At the beginning of rehab, I weighed 215 pounds on a good day and couldn't work ten feet without having chest pain and shortness of breath. Coupled with working out three times a week and not eating, I weighed 153 pounds. I know right, I was so proud of myself.

It was finally time for me to go to my follow-up appointment with Dr. Absi and Dr. Goel. I was excited to show them how well I was doing and how many changes I'd made in my lifestyle. Dr. Goel walked into the room said my name. The expression on his face was enough for me. He immediately went to find Dr. Absi, but he was stuck in OR performing surgery.

Two or three after my follow-up appointment, I started having full-body spasms. After reaching out to Dr. Basco, he told me to go to the emergency room. Even though I arrived at the Methodist Germantown in an ambulance, the nursing staff placed me against the wall screaming out in pain. One of the nurses named Jacqueline, checked my armband so she could test me for COVID-19. Even then, she placed me in a room that was the same size as a prison cell for me to wait. I was screaming out in pain for over two hours by myself because no family was allowed to accompany me.

It felt like it took forever for my test results to come back. I was screaming at the top of my lungs for at least two hours before someone stuck their head in the door to tell me why there was a delay. COVID had everything messed up. The same nurse came in tell let me know what I already knew. I was negative. She had fluids and everything she'd need to draw more blood. My body spasms more and more with each tube of blood she collects. After collected my blood sample, she was finally able to give me some Dilaudid.

 Within an hour, my results were back once again. My potassium was 1.2, magnesium 2.1, and hematocrit was critically low. What else could've gone wrong?

I couldn't help but think of how I'd made it through my fifth heart surgery to die from mineral depletion. I needed two blood and plasma transfusions and too many bags of fluids. It was like pulling teeth. The attendant on staff tried withholding my blood thinners because my INR/PTT levels were between 2.5 to 3.5. I tried telling

numerous times about my two mechanical valves. Dr. Tesmans was not happy when I challenged him. On the third day, my body was spasming again. I couldn't control my movements, and I was losing consciousness. I was so glad my oldest girl was able to stay with me that night. She ran to my bedside before yelling and screaming into the hallway. I couldn't speak or move again. My symptoms were the same as before. I could hear them talking to me, but I couldn't respond. The charge nurse Rian rushed into the room and by my bedside. Once I was stable, she asked if I needed anything.
I shook my head, "yes."
I forgot I had Dr. Absi's phone number on speed dial. I pointed over to the nightstand so someone could pass my cellphone. He answered on the third ring. I handed the phone to Molly to let her explain what was going on. He talked to them for almost thirty minutes when he hung up the phone. When my night nurse Tyana returned into the room, they Lovenox and Warfarin to get me regulated.

As much as I hate to use Lovenox, I didn't mind it because I had to be injected into my stomach. I could only imagine what he said, but whatever it was, it made them do their jobs.

My hematocrit, magnesium, potassium, and PTT/INR were back in range three days later.

Within a week, I was back to my old self and looking forward to going back to work.

My struggle with heart disease has not, nor will it ever be, a cakewalk, but I accept it. After I started wearing it on my sleeve, it became easier for me. Over the years, I've done my research and asked many questions, which allowed me to make better decisions regarding my life. I've made many mistakes along the way because I'm human, and that's the best way to learn. Please be adamant about your health.

My journal

Dear Char,

September 3rd is only a few days away, and I'm scared out of my mind. The only thing pulling me was thinking about is me not being to walk, talk, or breathe without being tired. I woke up this morning hoping my day would be a little better than yesterday, but as I tried to get out of my bed, it took everything in me to get out of it.

The first few days home were a blur. I remember laying in one spot, trying not to move a toe. The only times I got up were changing my dressings, rinse off, and using the bathroom. As I lay in bed unable to do anything for myself, the only thing I could think of doing to keep me sane was doing what I loved most, writing.
It may not seem like a lot to most people, but it helped me through. So here goes.

Day 5:
Today was a lot better than a few days before. This might sound cliche and worn out, but I truly have a great support system. From my husband DeWayne, my Mom. Mothers-in-law Gail and Bobbie, Cree, and everyone that calls and checks in me daily. Each day that I couldn't do much more than lay here, my husband brought his laptop and work downstairs into our bedroom with me. Each time I whimpered out in anguish, coughed, try to sneeze, DeWayne was right there. I have no idea how he differentiates between me trying to catch my breath,

wheezing, moaning, or crying when we slept at night, but each he pops up out of his sleep to make sure I am okay. I looked a hot mess, but he still kissed me and reassured me that I could make it through. Not to mention, I had to be at the doctor's office twice a week to get my INR level checked. With Covid running rampant worldwide, I was limited on how many could be at the Vanderbilt and during my checkups and appointments.

I can't lie. Laying in bed gave me a lot of time to reflect on all of the good and the not-so-good over that past year. My mindset after having surgery was different than before. I knew nothing was going to be the same after I recovered. There wasn't much I was afraid of anymore.

Dr. Absi made sure I knew there wasn't a lot of research or studies for patients with more than one mechanical heart valve. Because I'd decided to go through with the surgery, I'd have to monitor everything I ate and drank more than before for the rest of my life. I wish someone would have told me about the depression aspect of going under the knife for a life-threatening surgery. It wasn't that I didn't expect to go through it again. It's more so the fear of not making it. I've gone through four times before, but nothing of this magnitude. Again I found myself going through what most people would've turned down.

Who wants two mechanical valves clicking all day and night nonstop. I mean nonstop. Day6: When I woke this morning, I felt like recovery was going to be a breeze. My husband and father-in-law had gotten me a recliner for our bedroom. I was so excited I sat in the majority of the day. I was in pain, but I could hear Dr. Absi 's voice telling me not to get addicted to the opioids he'd given me. So I tried holding off taking anything extra until we made it home from getting my bloodwork done at AEL. By 10: 00, we were back at home, and everything from my throat done was hurting. If anyone was to ask, my pain level was way past ten. After making it back home, DeWayne made me get back in bed.

Day 7: OMG, I woke up in excruciating pain around 5:00 this morning. I yelled out in pain when I tried to rise up in bed without waking DeWayne up. He placed his hands on my thigh and made me wait for him. I'm not sure how or why I wrote this in the middle of the night, but I did.

Day 8: Progress is being made, I guess. This morning started a little different this morning. Before I could open my eyes, I was already awake. I felt invigorated mentally. I was ready to stretch, wash my face, butt, and brush my teeth. I prayed for my father to watch me from the heavenly skies. I prayed that he'd protect me from myself more than anything else. When I opened my eyes, my spirit relaxed even though every fiber in my being wished my Dad was standing next to me calling my name as he had many times before. I was surprised when I ran my hands up and down my chest, and it didn't hurt as it had before. Again progress. I stretched out my arms and legs as best as I could while lying in bed. I promise my recovery this time was

different, but I couldn't [ut my finger on how.
Everything was different, from the pain to the depression that went through multiple life-threatening heart surgeries. I had to learn how to walk, sit, eat, and drink all over again.
Day 9: I have to be honest with myself. Today felt different than yesterday to me. I've made it through another day, and I understand the trajectory of what I've gone through. I never knew the meaning of the old saying, " Don't judge a book by its cover, " until I started going through my journey with heart disease. I just needed to add a twist to it. Just because you can fit a person's shoes doesn't mean you can walk in them. Many people would've given up after surgery number two, but as I say often, I COULD NOT NOR WILL NOT GIVE UP ON ME. I WANT TO LIVE.
I laid in bed and allowed myself to cry, and with every tear that fell, I felt stronger.
There are times like this where I miss my Dad the most.

Day 10: It was 2 in the morning, and I was in so much pain. It was this that made me miss my Dad the most. I needed to hear him say, Babygirl, and it's going to be okay. Just hold on and be patient. Why in the hell does it hurt so bad. I belched, and I promise it felt like someone was stomping up and down my chest in steel-toe boots. Ughhhhhh, damn. My husband came rushing into the room when I called his name. He grabbed the Oxycocodone, Potassium, and my next dose of Torsemide. I tried my best not to bother him while working or in a meeting, and I'm unsure how he managed me and his job.

By 3:00, I was looking at my reflection in the mirror as if I were a stranger. How could I love myself when I didn't know who I was? At 5:00, I was lying in bed with DeWayne. I wonder if people knew love like I know love. After being with the same person for more than twenty years, you'd think that the love would fade away or things would change. But for me, my passion for DeWayne has grown stronger and deeper

with each day that passes. I love the look in his eyes when he looks at me. The way he thinks of me. The way he speaks to me. More than all of those things, I love the way he has learned to love me. I remember the day he came back into my life like it was yesterday. When we first started, I'd sit with my friends and family, and we'd talk about marriage. I never thought it would be him. I'd dream, but I could never see the face of the groom waiting for me at the altar. Some way, our conversation would go back to a man who finds a wife finds a good thing. My Mom would say that man knew he loved you and wanted to marry you when I was 15. He'd sit and talk to my Mom while I was at work, cheering at the basketball or football games.
Days 11 and 12 were too painful to write.

Day 13: I know I have to do more every day than before simply because moving around allows the heart to pump more easily and efficiently. My step count at midnight my step count was 2391. One thing going through this has taught me to be more vulnerable, even more so trusting. Even though DeWayne and I have been together for 23 years, it's hard to let go.

Day 14: It was two weeks (14 days) since I had surgery. I made it with two mechanical heart valves, which is unheard of. But now I'm a walking miracle, literally.
The hardest thing was going to be trying to get used to both of the valves clicking constantly. It was after midnight, and the sound was driving me crazy. DeWayne was upstairs playing the video game. It was the first night he'd gotten to do something other than taking care of me. There was no way I was going to bother him. I laid there and cried for almost thirty minutes. I cried not because I was hurting but because I'd made it through. My heart rate increased with each tear that fell from my eyes, making my pacemaker shock me.

Day 15: The most challenging part of today is listening to these valves clicking, clicking, and clicking.

I was up almost all of last night. Last night my heart kept skipping a beat, making my pacemaker shock me. It felt like I was a car with a stalling battery with the jumper cables attached. As I tried to calm myself, hoping my heart rate would regulate the pace of my heart, my heart started beating faster. Tears filled my eyes and traced my face. I laid there hoping and praying for the pain to go away. Before having surgery, I tolerated it better, but it was different because it was taken out of my chest and handled again. Because of the two mechanical valves, I have to learn how to manage the amount of Vitamin again. Even though I knew I couldn't risk forming a blood clot, it didn't make me feel any better.

Day 18: Oh, how glad I am. My body is trying to heal itself in more than one. I have more energy, my range of motion is started to improve, and it puts a smile on my face was my chest isn't crackling every time I move. It's hard as hell for me to shake the hospital hours.]After being in the hospital for almost two weeks, my sleep schedule was thrown off.

Despite the visible scars, I still try to cover up. When we go out, I still hold my head high and plaster a smile on my face. I constantly repeat, "I still had my head high because despite my circumstances," I'm still a queen, and as Maya Angelou says, still I rise.

What does is it mean exactly?

I rise out of this bed even my chest crackles, and the pain rises from my chest, stomach, and sternum. I rise out of my chair because I know sitting there will allow unwanted self-doubt and depression to consume me. I have to start some type of exercise. I knew from experience I had to start small. I made up a plan. Today, I must up and walked from my recliner and into the hallway. Tomorrow, I'd try to make it from our master bedroom to the living room at least twice a day this week and gradually add on. I'd do this until I started rehab.

I know better than most if I allow myself to sir and not fight for my life, depression would only worsen, which will allow the excess fluid to fill my lungs and turn into pneumonia.

I wrote myself a note and placed it on my bedside table. It said, "Charnique is strong, resilient, beautiful, kind, courageous, wise, encouraging, and intelligent, and most of all, you are a FIGHTER. I could've given up years ago. Instead, I choose my life.

Day 19: This morning, the pain in my neck was worse, so I laid in bed for almost a full hour with the heating pad on it. I could've gotten out of bed when DeWayne came in so I could take a shower, but instead, I laid back down until almost noon. My throat was still a problem, but I was hungry as hell. DeWayne used Uber Eats for the first time because he'd be in meetings most of the day. I had a small amount of past, two broccoli florets, 1/4 o the salmon he'd gotten. Once I was sure DeWayne was out of the room, I snuck into the bathroom and tried and put on a little bit of makeup. As I turned around to head back to the recliner, I heard DeWayne's voice. Oh my Gosh, he was mad as hell. He fussed for almost ten minutes about me possibly hurting myself. I agreed and sat back down for about an hour.

After taking a nap, I was up and back at it. I got out of my chair and started walking in place at a steady pace while I watched A Different World. I surprised myself. I wanted to be out of bed so bad I came up with a routine. My mother inlaw called at 2:30 to see what I wanted for dinner. I wanted some tacos, and I determined to be out of my bedroom when she started cooking.

Day 20: I am happy and so proud of myself. Before my mother-in-law got home with everything we needed to cook, I'd taken me something for pain. I was ready. I had Cam bring the Bluetooth speaker into the kitchen. I made my way into the kitchen when she started browning the meat. Gail asked what in the hell I was out of the bed but at the same time happy I was going to keep her company. I'm not sure if I ook over the kitchen or just sat down when she saw me pedaling away on the veggies. I cook everything. Earlier, DeWayne let me go outside to harvest. He only let me out for ten minutes, which was long enough to grab fresh jalapenos, bell peppers, cilantro, and tomatoes. This morning after walking in place, I had 3287 steps, and by the time I finished making dinner, I had over 7,000. After showering and getting my blood drawn, I was in pain and tired as hell. Fall had officially begun, leaves were falling, and the birds were chirping away. I loved being out on the patio writing or typing away on my laptop. It has been a different smell in the air that brought a particular type of calm over me. On our way home, DeWayne picked up Tokyo Grill for lunch. When we made it home, I finally sat in my favorite place in my living room, my oversized chair with my laptop. I stayed there almost the entire day until my chest started hurting at about 8 o'clock.

Day 21: I have cooties. I'm going back to bed.

Day 22: Nyquil is the best. Yesterday I woke up feeling as I had caught a cold. I still couldn't cough without hurting myself, even when pressing my cardiac pillow against my chest. Omg, I can't believe I hadn't spoken of my pillow. Well, anytime a patient undergoes heart surgery, the hospital usually provides them with a patient designed by their cardiac team. I use mine anytime I stand, sit down, sneeze, cough, and anytime my sternum starts to shift. I like to think I'm a veteran. Instead of waking my husband up in the middle of the night, I use my abdominal muscles and legs. Don't judge me. It has worked thus far. This time it took me about three for the incisions to heal in the pelvic area.

Day 23: I slept the majority of the day. I was so happy when I got out of the shower. The surgical tape had started coming off. I was already self-conscious about all of the scars on my forehead, neck, stomach, and thighs. UGH...

Day 24: Today's my Dad's birthday, and more than anything in this world, I wish I could see his face. I'm not sure how long I laid perfectly still talking to my Dad. I promise I could see his face smiling at me. I asked for his protection and strength to carry me through my storm. When I opened my eyes, I was ready to face whatever was in my way. When I got out of bed, I felt refreshed and renewed. I painted a smile on my face.

Day 25: I waited for DeWayne to go up the stairs since he was working from home. I woke up when the alarm went off with DeWayne. I feel great. Last night I surprised DeWayne and myself when I made it the steps by myself. I didn't have any chest pain or out of breath. Whoop, whoop, that spirometer is working. While I was downstairs, I could hear him rapping and making beats. He stopped when he saw me standing behind him. The smile on his face made my heart sing. I grabbed as tight as he could hug me without hurting me. I could tell he was just as happy as I was. After sitting down beside him, he played a track that made me cry. He'd made a song for me and how strong I was. He said my strength made him stronger. I could not stop the tears from running down my face. The song was beautiful.

Day 26: I was up at 4:00 this morning. I knew if I'd gotten out of bed, my dogs would have gotten up, waking up everybody in the house, including my husband. So I laid there watching one of my childhood favorite TV shows, The Jeffersons until I fell back asleep.

Day 27: I yeah, I feel great this morning. I got up and snuck into the shower while DeWayne was upstairs on a conference call. Girl, I feel so good. I was finally able to wet my hair and pull it back into a ponytail. When I got out of the shower and looked at my reflection hated what I saw. Even though I know every scar I have has allowed me to still be here instead of buried inside the grave. It didn't stop the tears from falling from my eyes. I stood still at that moment. I needed every tear to fall from my eyes to give me strength. The surgical tape was almost entirely off, but my sternum was swollen and hurting like hell. Day 28: I can't believe it's almost been a month since I'd had surgery. We were up bright and early and out of the house around 4:00 this morning, so we'd be o time for my appointment at Vanderbilt. My appointment with Dr. Absi went very well. When he came into the exam room, Dr. Absi said, "Charnique, is that you"? OMg, you look great. At the end of the appointment, he got my husband's attention and "I told you I would give you your wife back to you. Looking at me, both of them smiled at me. That was encouraging. He was so proud of his work he came back into the room with a few of

his surgical nurses. Dr. Absi said, " look at her. She looks different, doesn't she?
Days 30 through 31: I had to rest after riding in the car for almost 7 hours.

I made it one whole month, yes.

Day 32: I'm feeling better than I have in years. It's time for me to make some changes mentally, physically, and emotionally.
I'm so amazed by how good I feel and so soon. If Dr. Jerry Gooch had done his job correctly, I wouldn't have endured all of the shortness of breath, palpitations, dizziness, or chest pain. But he was more concerned with how many surgeries he could perform daily instead of the wellbeing of his patients. I can only imagine where I would be I didn't have to put my life on hold. Hell, I may have been able to finish nursing school.
As they say, everything happens for a reason. Going through five surgeries humbled me and made me grow into

myself. I learned to love myself and to choose myself first.

Day 33: I messed up and let my Potassium and Magnesium drop critically low. I feel like crap. I'm just happy my body hadn't started spasming. My weight is still dropping off, and I'm so excited. I need my head to stop throbbing. DeWayne came in to check on me for a few minutes. He wanted me to get some rest but wanted us to go for a light walk just to see how far I've come.

I just woke up, and it was a little after 3:00. I fell brand new. After pulling myself, I could feel someone looking at me. I knew it couldn't be anyone but DeWayne. He had the biggest smile on his face. I should have known he was up to something. As soon as he turned the corner, I could see the white styrofoam cup in his hand.

I looked at him for confirmation, potassium?

DeWayne smiled again and said yes.

God knows this is some horrible mess to drink. I had to take 120meq. That mess burned my throat and my stomach. I complained for ten minutes straight even though I knew he wasn't going to back down. It had practically become our routine three times a day. But dang it, I had to double my dose if I didn't want to go to the hospital.

About an hour later, I was up and headed to take a shower to put on some clothes. While I waited for DeWayne to finish his last meeting for the day, I snuck outside to check on my garden. Luckily it was October, so my veggies hadn't frozen. I had my scissors and little bucket.

I loved being outside. The last time I was outside looking at my garden, DeWayne didn't allow me to pick much. I couldn't believe how much had grown. I was sad when I saw my watermelon. It was about the size of an heirloom tomato before it'd gone bad. I was able to pick cucumbers, tomatoes, zucchini, bell peppers, carrots, jalapenos, ghost peppers, Thai peppers, reaper peppers, and banana peppers. That was enough for me.

Day 34: We got out this morning, and I soaked up every minute of it up. I feel awesome.

Day 35: If I weren't constipated, I say I feel great. When I got up this morning to use the bathroom and shower, I had a trial of blood trailing. DeWayne and I went for a walk, and I walked two blocks up and back, which in my mind is four blocks. Hahaha.

Day 36: I can't wait to make it six weeks. I can't believe it. Tears are running down my face as I type this. I am so grateful. DeWayne may not know it yet, but I'm fixing my breakfast after I shower. I feel great, and I need to take some of the stress off of him. As soon as I hear him in one of his meetings, I will wash a load of clothes and hopefully straighten up the house. Note to self, girl, you did just that. I'm so proud of you.

Day 36: It is officially six weeks from the day I was admitted to the hospital at Vanderbilt. I feel so good. After showering, I went straight to the kitchen to see what I could cook for dinner. Shocking myself, I prepped everything for lunch and dinner. I soaked the chicken in vinegar and salt to pull all of the excess blood and bacteria out. Cut the potatoes so I could make mashed potatoes, chopped veggies, and made sandwiches for lunch.

By 6:30, I was ready. I had Molly find me some music to listen to. I fried the chicken, and everything was history. My husband didn't think I saw him, but how could I miss it with a head as big as his how could I miss it. He was trying to be funny after getting settled back into my recliner to rest. I wrote, "WRITE YOUR TRUTH."

Stopping allowing what other people may think or react. No one can tell your truth better than you.

Take your time relearning what you may have forgotten.

Day 43: Living with heart disease makes me appreciate the simplest things. After going through open-heart surgery again, I look forward to smelling my DeWayne's cologne when I wake up in recovery. I'm still not sure how but smelling his cologne calms me when he's near. There's one thing he and I always go back to, which is when I'd lost a lot of blood, my surgical team wasn't sure if I'd live or not. I was in ICU, my vitals had dropped, and despite their best efforts, nothing was working.

As he walked into the room and sat beside me in my hospital bed, my vitals started improving. When I woke up, he was there. The nurse working on me that day told me everything. From the look on his face when they told him I wasn't doing well to him sitting by my bedside watching Sports Center on a TV that shouldn't be in the room.

Day 46: I'm going to do things my way.

Day 47: Oh my god, to say this has been the most challenging hurdle for me to push through. I'm praying with every fiber in my body that I could go more than five years without me having to go through it again. I pray the 5th time is a Charm.

It's been almost 12 weeks. I can't believe it's been three months. My support system thus far has been incredible. I can't stop the tears from falling down my face, and I'm not sure if I want to. I know a lot of people would've given up and stopped trying, but that's not me. I'll never stop trying to live. Oh, before I forget, I started physical therapy Monday. My team is so patient with me. After doing my assessment, I told them I've been through PT before, which made it much more manageable. They worked the heck of me, but I enjoyed each moment because I knew what my result would be.

Day 49: I felt kind of bad when I woke up this morning. As much as I hate to take potassium, I knew from the way I thought I needed to take a double dose if I planned on going to therapy this morning. So I peeled myself out the door and headed into the kitchen. Lookie, lookie, lookie. DeWayne's butt was standing at the island, pouring orange juice and three potassium effervescent tablets into a cup.

As I looked into the mirror after showering, I looked at myself in the mirror and promised myself to use this time to write my book and strengthen myself more before I had to go back to work.

I know if I'm still working with the person, it would be more stressful than before I left on leave. I followed my advice as used her as my motivation to lose weight and get stronger. I promise you before I went out on FMLA leave, she and I almost fought in the pharmacy. During our argument, I was running on nothing more than adrenaline. After my supervisor got us to shut up, I had chest pain, my head was tired, and I could barely breathe.

I said all of that to say one thing and one thing only. I wish people would stop thinking only about themselves and what the next person was doing. "Just because you can fit your foot inside my size eight shoe, that doesn't mean you can walk in them." I was happy as hell when Dr. Absi called and scheduled my surgery date. After finishing my fifth week of rehab, I jumped into the shower and onto my scale. I couldn't believe the scale when I looked down. It read 157. I stepped off and back on to be sure I was reading it wrong. Nope, 157 it is. I'd lose over 57 pounds.

September 1, 2021: I can't believe I've made almost a full year. Girl, you made. Marking it through yet another open-heart surgery proves just how strong you are. I love you, and don't give up
Love me.

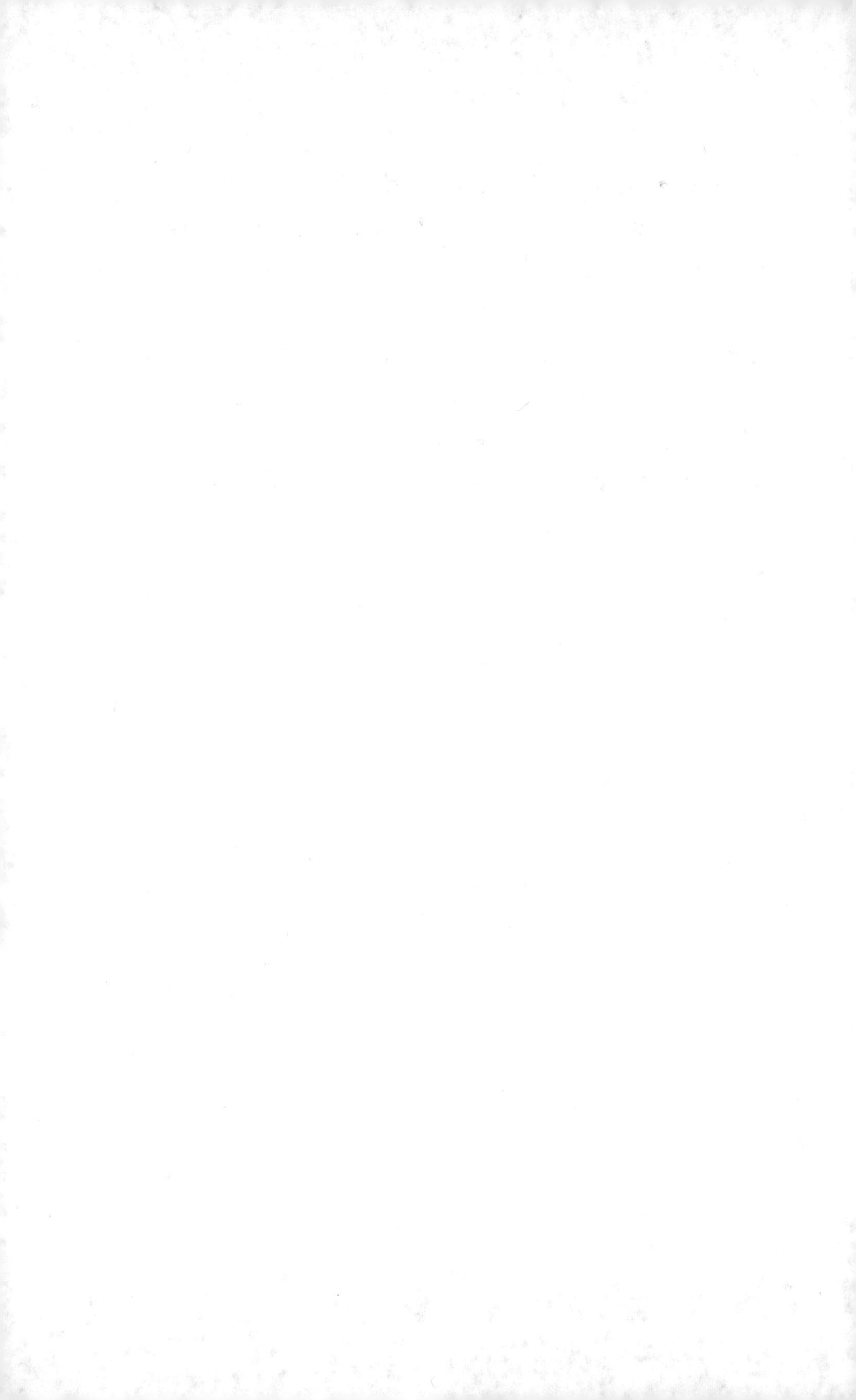

www.ingramcontent.com/pod-product-compliance
Lightning Source LLC
Chambersburg PA
CBHW061337250726
48657CB00004B/1202